Sick
Idiot

by

ASHLEY BOYNES-SHUCK

Sick Idiot

Disclaimer:

This book is nonfiction. However, some names and/or identifying details may have been changed to protect the privacy of individuals. I have tried to recreate events, locales, and conversations from my memories of them. This book is not intended as a substitute for the medical advice of physicians. The reader should regularly consult a physician in matters relating to his/her health and particularly with respect to any symptoms that may require diagnosis or medical attention.

To contact the author, please email: author.abshuck@gmail.com

Cover Photography and Design Copyright © 2015
by Matthew Shuck of Shuck Photography

Styling by Kristen Varoli of Contempo Artistries Salon

A portion of proceeds from this book sale will go to charity.

DEDICATION

This book is dedicated to all of you who live with chronic or invisible illness. I dedicate it to the folks who are striving to get a diagnosis, and to the warriors who have been living with an illness or disability for years. This is for all of you who choose to thrive and survive despite health problems, who keep smiling even when times are difficult, and for everyone, whether you're healthy or not, who has ever felt different or had a "Sick Idiot" moment of their own.

CONTENTS

GRATITUDE &
ACKNOWLEDGMENTS

First and foremost, I need to thank God for — well, everything! — but particularly for bestowing this wonderful opportunity upon me, and for placing both the desire to write <u>and</u> a sense of humor within my heart. I would like to take a moment to thank my awesome husband, Michael Shuck, who has truly been by my side through sickness and in (rare occasions of) health. (And who, upon hearing my idea for this book, suggested that I use my phrase, "Sick Idiot" as the title!) I also need to thank my loving parents, Sharon and Rick Boynes, who have always encouraged me to not let my health problems define who I am. They have taught me by example what true strength and hard work look like. They, along with my husband, family, pets, and friends, have shown me unconditional love — the kind of love that I aim to show towards others.

I want to thank my grandparents, Nana and Bups (a.k.a. Eileen and Leon Louis,) and Grandma (Joan) Boynes, as well as my late Grandpap (Bob) Boynes. Grandma, you have been a true picture of strength and fortitude through hardship. Nana, you have shown me how to handle illness with grace … and good style! Bups, you were my all-star coach, and are an all-star grandfather, too. Grandpap Boynes, you're my guardian angel who has helped me through many a tough time. I'd like to acknowledge my brother Ryan Boynes and my soon-to-be sister-in-law, Meghan Flick. You guys continually inspire me and make me proud, and I thank you for all of your support. By proxy, I'd like to, in part, dedicate this to the memory of your best friend, Curtis Valent, who I mention in this book.

To all of my dear girlfriends, Kristen Varoli, Valerie Moore, Hadley Kappers, Nicole Sichak, Sara Andreen, Caroline McPherson, Valerie Spanovich, Christina Gomez, Eileen Allan, and so many more, as well as to my cousin-and-built-in-bestie Jacquie Lyon, and all of my other friends, you are amazing examples of strong, beautiful women who I respect, admire, and treasure. Thanks for always being there for me. I want to say thank you, also, to my in-laws, aunts, uncles, and cousins, who have always supported and encouraged me through the years. You uplift me, and I am proud and grateful to know you and to have the chance to love you.

I'd like to acknowledge all who follow me as Arthritis Ashley online, and give a thank you to all of my "rheum mates" and "spoonie pals" who help lessen the burden of life with chronic illness on a daily basis through your kind words and inspiring stories. I would like to thank and acknowledge the Arthritis Foundation, the American

College of Rheumatology, Healthline.com, and the people of Crossroads United Methodist Church in North Fayette, PA, particularly the women of my Small Group. Thank you to the doctors in my life who have taken the time to care: Dr. Charles Pucevich, Dr. David Binion, Dr. Bobak Robert Mozayeni, Dr. Josef Tybl, Dr. Paul Gardner, Dr. Evgeniy Shchelchkov, Dr. Gabrielle Bonhomme, Dr. Frank Verri, and Dr. Viorica Crisan, plus the many doctors and nurses who I've dealt with in passing during various hospital stays. Thank you to all in the medical profession who show care, compassion, patience, respect, and kindness. Thank you to everyone who puts patients first, and thank you to anyone is working towards a cure.

Thank you to Lindsey Smith, Joshua Rosenthal, and the Institute for Integrative Nutrition for inspiring me to write this book, to David Martin and Lisa Mauti for believing in my work as an arthritis advocate, to Matthew Shuck of Shuck Photography for the photography and cover design, to Kristen Varoli of Contempo Artistries Salon for doing my hair and makeup for the cover and countless other times, to Kathi Shuck for allowing us to shoot in Kathi's Dance Studio, and to Lilliput Doll Hospital for giving my Winnie the "brain surgery" that she needed.

Lastly, I have to extend lots of love, wags, purrs, and hugs to my "fur-babies," who constantly fill my heart with joy and make me smile ... even on my biggest Sick Idiot days.

INTRODUCTION: WHY "SICK IDIOT?"

Before the PC-Police start a petition to boycott my book because of its mildly controversial title that could seem seemingly-derogatory towards the chronically ill, let me explain ...

It was your average weekday. I, however, was having trouble doing average things. It was a day like many others, a day I wasn't feeling well. As Murphy's Law would have it, anything that could happen, did happen. I overslept, my knee locked up, I had swollen glands, and swollen hands. I couldn't open a jar. I could barely open the refrigerator. My dog knocked me over, and I had a migraine that would cause a grown man to bawl like a newborn.

Simply put, it just wasn't my day. I had it up to my aching neck with bad news, pain, sickness, and rain. The frustration mounted, and my usual "positive and smiling" facade was melting away with each new "damn it!" and "what now?" that the day threw my way.

By the time my husband got home from work, I had what some would call a nutty. Insert your word of choice: tantrum, meltdown, hysteria, whatever. The point is that it was not pretty. I went on and on about how awful my day

was, and how icky I felt, only to unexpectedly announce
(with dramatic exclamation):

"I'm nothing but a Sick Idiot!"

Well, for whatever reason, that random proclamation
caused the first smile of my day. My husband and I burst
into laughter while I wiped away those nagging tears. My
sobs dissolved into a fit of giggles, and as he folded me
into his arms, I felt just a bit better about life.

There is most certainly nothing funny about being sick,
so you may be wondering what's funny about me calling
myself a Sick Idiot. For one, I don't use the word idiot
very often. Secondly, one does not typically call a sick
person an idiot. Lastly, I'm not an idiot at all. I'm actually a
member of the high-IQ society Mensa, and am, by many
testing standards, considered an actual genius, or at the
very least, gifted. (This fact surprises people sometimes. I
don't know if I can blame them.)

For such a childish choice of words to so forcefully
erupt from my blubbering lips was pretty hilarious. It was
obvious that I was just having a "woe-is-me" moment,
complete with the crossed arms and eye rolls of a petulant
child. I didn't stomp my feet — but I could have, both for
emphasis and to better complete my frazzled,
embarrassing tantrum.

Overall, it's just not like me. I don't call people idiots. I
don't whine and cry about my multitudinous health
problems. I don't stomp my feet, or complain about the
plethora of rotten cards I've been dealt. I just saddle up

and soldier on. I try to stay happy, positive, grateful, and friendly.

To be fair, being sick sucks. But, I usually attempt to embrace it — I try to turn negatives into positives, find my strength through my suffering, make my burden my blessing, my mess my message, and all that jazz. I usually just march onward and upward. I get through it.

Yet, every so often, due to the whole "being sick sucks" thing, I may have a little nutty. We warmly refer to these moments as my "Sick Idiot" moments. It applies to a lot of other things, too. Medical bill? Gotta budget the Sick Idiot money. Friends inviting me to run a 5K? Can't, I'm a Sick Idiot. Husband coming home to a total hot mess? Better text him a warning: "I'm in Sick Idiot-mode today." I think even healthy folks can have "Sick Idiot" moments. If you've fallen down the steps, immediately had to shower because someone sneezed on you in the checkout line of the supermarket, gotten chicken pox on your school photo day, or wore a cast in your wedding photo, you, my friend, are welcomed warmly into the club of Sick Idiots. If you've even just had one of those days where everything went wrong and you had a full-scale meltdown, then you've probably experienced your own Sick Idiot moment or two.

It may not be politically correct, or even all that cute or catchy, but, to me, it's at least a little bit funny to call my not-so-healthy alter-ego a big, fat, sick, idiot. As you'll see in the coming pages, I think that humor and a positive perspective are essential prescriptions to treat all that ails you in life. After all, laughter is the best medicine, right? Sick or not, I hope you'll enjoy my funny little health memoir — all of which is, for better or for worse, 100%

3

true. This is my sometimes-sucky, sometimes-funny, often-inspiring, and always-blessed journey through life as a chronically ill (but still pretty fabulous) woman.

So, turn the page, and limp with me as we travel through my life as a Sick Idiot.

THE SICK LIST:
MY ENDLESS DIAGNOSES

Before we go any further, here is a list all of the conditions I've been diagnosed with over the years. Hopefully, knowing what all I have dealt with will give you a better perspective and some helpful background as you read my ridiculous but true stories. Here we go:

- Polyarticular Juvenile Idiopathic Arthritis and Adult-Onset Rheumatoid Arthritis
- Celiac Disease with Villous Atrophy
- Lupus (SLE and drug-induced)
- Sjögren's Syndrome
- Chiari Malformation
- Mixed Connective Tissue Disease
- Chronic Systemic Migraines
- Osteoarthritis
- Osteopenia
- Pernicious Anemia
- Tarsal Coalition
- Chronic Tinnitus with Upper-Register Hearing Loss
- Idiopathic Myopathy
- Acute Gastroparesis and Gastritis
- Vitiligo
- Tenia Versicolor
- Bull's Eye Maculopathy
- Supraventricular Tachycardia

- Sinus Tachycardia & POTS (Postural Orthostatic Tachycardia Syndrome)
- Hypotension
- Generalized Immunodeficiency
- Chronic Muscle Spasms & Neuropathy
- Spondyloarthropathy
- Polymyositis
- Palindromic Rheumatism
- Gastroesophageal Reflux Disease
- Bile Reflux Syndrome
- Chronic Sinusitis
- Dermatofibroma
- Sialolithiasis (Wharton's Stone)
- Fibrocystic Breast Disease
- Costochondritis
- Autoimmune Iritis
- Bell's Palsy
- Mild Scoliosis
- Spinal Rotation
- Cervical Spinal Lordosis
- Fibromyalgia
- Thyroid Imbalance
- Multiple Chemical Sensitivities/Idiopathic Environmental Intolerance/Allergies (Like, allergic to everything.)
- Various Cysts, Nodules, and Dysplasias

One doctor even told me I had "Spina Bifida Occulta," but no one else has ever corroborated that, so we'll leave that one out for now. But ... yeah. This, my friends, is where the "sick" in Sick Idiot comes from.

THAT TIME I WAS BORN A
DISASTER WAITING TO HAPPEN

The only time in my life that I was ever early for anything was the day I was born.

On September 29th, 1983, I came into this world at about four whole whopping pounds, five weeks before I was due. I guess you could say that I've been surprising people and keeping them guessing from day one.

I've always had a knack for being different. Even now, at 31 years old, I am constantly reminded, day in and day out, that I'm different from most of my peers. A sinus infection could knock me down for two months. I can't wear the high heels that I love, and, for me, ordering at a restaurant causes more than your average case of menu anxiety. Carrying my purse for any extended period of time hurts my shoulders, and I panic at church when I'm encouraged to shake hands with strangers, because I have to be concerned about germs. I also worry about being judged at some churches when I cannot kneel for extended periods of time. I can't simply join a softball league for fun, or commit to bowling plans on the weekend, because I don't know in advance how my body will behave. If your child has a cold, I have to be leery about hugging not just them, but you, as well. The perfume section of Macy's is a danger zone. Fluorescent lighting is a migraine trigger. Standing for too long, sitting for too long, walking for too long, being on the computer for too long: all of these things are sometimes hard for me. My weight fluctuates less from exercise and nutrition, and more so from medications. Healthcare headlines are not just background noise to me: they are news that matters and has a very real impact on my life. I can't sign up for a race on a whim, or eat something without reading the ingredient list. I am used to people staring when I limp, and I'm used to missing out on things because of my health. I feel that living with health issues forces me to have less free time to work with, because so much of my free time is spent being sick. My healthy time is limited. Every decision I make is somehow based on my health and my body. I'm different, but I'm used to it.

Despite being different, and despite being a preemie, I was seemingly healthy and happy as a baby. Some moments that stand out in my childhood memories relate to my health, much like they do as an adult. I remember getting pneumonia in kindergarten and having to stay home from school. I hated it. I loved school and have always suffered from the affliction called FOMO, or, Fear of Missing Out.

I got a taste of what life with illness would be like, too, when a random shelf-falling-on-head incident caused a potential concussion that led me to have to sit out of a t-ball game. Watching from the sidelines, I learned early on, wasn't fun. Little did I know, I'd have to get used to it.

But when you're a kid, you don't think about these things too much. Sure, it stinks in the moment to be kept home from school or to have to miss a t-ball game, but when you're five years old, you don't realize that you could end up feeling like you're on the sidelines for your entire life. That is what's great about being a kid: innocence.

I also remember two different occasions where I was bitten by ticks in my early years of elementary school. I often played in the woods, was always outdoors, had dogs, and went camping, so it wasn't that absurd of a notion to find a tick here and there, particularly given the fairly rural area where I'd grown up. Did these tick bites cause my lifelong propensity towards autoimmune and rheumatic illness? We'll never know. What I do know is that a lot began to unfold in the years to follow, but, despite having dealt with illness since I was very young, I had a wonderful childhood and have had a wonderful life. Different doesn't always mean bad. It may not have been normal, but it was *my* normal.

THAT TIME I GOT PUSHED DOWN THE STEPS AND CONTRACTED GROWING PAINS

The day began innocently enough. In fact, it was about as pure and innocent as you could get: it was the day of my First Holy Communion. I, decked out in my all-white gown complete with lace and bows and frills, was beyond excited to rock my bun and my veil through the church like a miniature bride.

Naturally, I was also excited because there was going to be a big party for me afterwards. The actual Communion went fine, and was about as exciting and eventful as any First Holy Communion mass at a Catholic church. There were only 8 of us making Communion that day, so it went rather quickly, but I recall that swallowing the Communion wafer couldn't have gone quickly enough.

I had always been somewhat envious of the adults who got to go up for Communion each mass, and was disappointed to find that the Eucharist tasted less like a divine treat and more like parchment paper. I actually remember thinking that it tasted the way that fish food smelled, and I wondered if my fish were equally disappointed.

After the obligatory church photos, it was party time. I couldn't have been more pumped for my special day. All I knew is that I'd get chicken wings, cake, presents, and cards. It seemed to me like a bonus birthday party, complete with an extra-fancy dress and many guests whom I didn't really know.

Among these mystery guests was a child. This child wasn't a direct relative of mine, but he was there. Being a 2nd grader, I, of course, paired up with the girls. We went our separate ways, away from said guest and the other boys, probably off playing with my Barbies or examining my beautiful dress. The boys were wild, getting yelled at every five minutes to stop running in the house, to quiet down, or to quit throwing things.

I was one of those girly-girls who also had a major tomboy side. A part of me actually preferred running around with the boys, playing kickball, Nintendo, and Teenage Mutant Ninja Turtles. But my affinity towards roughhousing with the guys is what led to an injury that may have set off a chain of events that would eventually change my life.

This is where Mystery Guest came into play. Now, I don't recall the specifics: remember, I was only 8 years old. What I do recall, though, is a little boy pushing me down the steps. I, in my ruffles of white, tumbled down the stairs, head over heels, or, as my dad once said, "ass over teakettle," landing squarely on my ankle.

The exact timeline is murky, but at some point I ended up at the hospital for the first time of many. It could have been that night; it could have been the next day. I could call my mother and ask, but the detail seems too minute to bother. At any rate, there I was: this tiny little thing, skinny, with lanky limbs and tanned skin, observing the hospital with wary curiosity and the innocent optimism that comes with being an 8-year-old. I don't remember being scared, just curious. It almost seemed like an adventure to me, so other than the ankle pain, the experience of being a the hospital didn't register as "negative." (Boy, how things would change.)

My big brown eyes watched the nurses bustling about, observed the other patients in the waiting room, and impatiently flipped through a *Highlights* magazine. Once they called us into the examination room, I bravely put on my oversized hospital gown. Drowning in the hideous garb, I followed a lady in blue scrubs to a room with lots of metal machinery. She explained that I'd be getting an x-ray, and I nodded politely — again, not scared, just curious. I wondered how this camera could take a picture of my bones that were inside of me.

As I lay still for the images, I thought about bones. The kids at school called me Ashley Bones. It was just too easy: my last name was Boynes, and I was a bony little thing: thin and all limbs. I wondered how funny it would be to them if Ashley Bones had Broken Bones, but I figured that Ashley Bones was better than my other nickname at school: Ashley Beaver-Bucktooth Boynes.

Let me be clear: I never had buckteeth, per se. I had big front teeth — like a cute little bunny. But they didn't stick out. I wasn't a beaver. I should also state that while I knew I had these nicknames floating around, and was called "big-eyed vanilla ice cream" by an African American student in kindergarten, I wasn't bullied (yet) to the point of emotional anguish of any sort. In fact, the year before all of this, my "playing with the boys" got me into trouble at school the first time when a friend's mom called my first-grade teacher to let her know that I was punching her son at recess. I learned my lesson, though, and am proud to say that I never again was a bully or a fighter. Violence is never the answer.

Neither was pushing a little girl down the steps, but Mystery Guest apparently missed that memo, and there I was, awaiting x-ray results. The doctor came in, and all I understood was that I needed crutches and an Air Cast. I was kind of disappointed that I didn't get a *real* cast: it always was fun to sign other kids' casts and draw doodles on them. I got a weirdo cast: a kind that no one else at school had ever worn. I was not a happy camper.

The crutches hurt my armpits, and I felt embarrassed about the whole thing. I do remember how nice it was to have kids at school eagerly volunteering to carry my books. I don't remember being teased any more than usual, and life went on.

In fact, life went on for a couple of years without incident. That time I got pushed down the steps was all but a memory. The only problem was that the physical pain simply wouldn't go away — it lingered, like a houseguest who simply won't leave, or a zit during prom week, or the frustration we've all felt from the series finale of *Lost*. I didn't really tell anyone about it. I continued life as usual: reading my *Babysitters Club* and *Sweet Valley High* books, watching Nickelodeon and the Disney Channel after school, practicing for and winning the spelling bee, and writing short stories in my GATE class. There were also sports and physical activities that I loved. I played softball and basketball. I enjoyed gym class (particularly bowling days and the shuttle run part of the Presidential Physical Fitness Tests!) I liked playing kickball, Capture the Flag, and Release with friends; I liked hiking through the woods with my cousins; I adored bike riding at my family's camp in Ohio; I liked making up dances and doing my Barbie & Paula Abdul aerobics videos with my girlfriends from school.

But, it was during this era that I would truly realize that I was a little bit different from my friends. I wasn't able to run well during basketball practice — my ankle always hurt, and it slowed me down. I noticed that I always had to crack my wrists, that I was tired a lot, that I got sick easily, and that I would be sore after softball games, whereas others would not be — at least, not to the same level.

We went to a few different pediatricians who told my parents that I was experiencing growing pains. That was that, growing pains it was. I suppose the link between my tumble down the steps and these new "growing pains" was not apparent at the time. So I focused on designing outfits for my dolls and crushing on JTT from *Home Improvement* and Justin Timberlake from *the Mickey Mouse Club*. Life would go on, and I would experience many growing pains, as many other kids my age would do. The only difference is that my growing pains were physical, and actually painful. And, again like the *Lost* finale, we had no real answers at all.

THAT TIME I CRIED ON THE PITCHER'S MOUND AND SAW MY GRANDMA'S DOCTOR

My softball team became family to me. In fact, my grandfather Bups and mom were among the team's coaches, so the aforementioned statement is partially literal. The girls on the team became my close friends on and off the field. We were sure we'd be BFFAE (best friends for ever and ever!) and we were bonded by hazy late-summer practices at Morgan Field and the unique smell of a new leather ball glove and Big League Chew bubble gum.

The sound of the ball cracking off the bat against the backdrop of cheers and the smell of french fries became an addiction to me. I lived, ate, slept, and breathed softball. I couldn't get enough of the adrenaline that flowed through my sometimes-tempestuous-and-always-competitive veins as I stepped up to bat (often being cleanup batter, *thankyouverymuch*,) or as I stepped onto the mound in the bottom of the 9th.

There weren't many better feelings than those of striking a batter out, or hitting a home run or grand slam. There's nothing quite like getting a trophy for actually winning instead of simply participating, and not much beats being invited to an All-Stars team. I am lucky that I got to experience all of those things. But, as you'll see in stories to come, when it comes to me, there are always really high highs, and really low lows. I'm the yin-yang personified, a Libra at her finest: the good is balanced with bad, and vice versa.

So, it is fitting that my many years as a ball player, from t-ball up to slow-pitch and then fast-pitch softball, were tainted with some not-so-great moments. I would suffer indescribable pain after games or practices — pain that I would, for a long time, keep secret. I noticed that my hands would hurt when I was writing at school. I got headaches all the time. My shoulder, knee, and ankle killed me after basketball or softball games.

As an elementary school student, I was borrowing my dad's Ben-Gay ointment and taking Tylenol for pain. While I was having a blast with school and sports, I often felt generally unwell. After talking with my aunt, who is a nurse and who would ironically later be diagnosed with RA herself, my parents decided that I should see a specialist. "Growing pains," as it turns out, are not really a thing that people of my age would have continued to experience. Some doctors deny the existence of growing pains at all, but when they do seem to occur, they are typically seen in children ages 4-6 years of age. So, even when I was first diagnosed with them, I was nine years old and well past the typical age of onset. Additionally, growing pains don't typically tend to hang out throughout a kid's entire life, so, there's that.

My maternal grandma, Nana, has rheumatoid arthritis, and one of the types of specialists on our list to possibly see was a rheumatologist. So, we made an appointment with her doctor. My first trip there was unnerving; I was easily the youngest there, by a good 50 or 60 years. Even to this day, I feel awkward in his waiting room, where most of the other patients have graying hair, wrinkled skin, and perms, as I play on my iPhone, often with a visible tattoo or two, and fun colorful streaks in my hair. I don't exactly fit in at the rheumatologist, and I never have.

During that first visit, I was quiet. My mom did a lot of the talking, and she and my doctor discussed me like I wasn't in the room. I didn't mind; I liked looking at the posters and the life-sized model of the human knee. After a lot of blood work, x-rays, and physical exams, I was eventually diagnosed with polyarticular juvenile rheumatoid arthritis, now known as juvenile idiopathic arthritis. I was about 10 years old, going on 11, and I had arthritis. I was also advised to quit sports.

My heart sank. There was no way that I was going to do that. So, I continued to play softball. Then, it happened: The Defining Event.

I call it The Defining Event because, I believe that it was the particular moment when the JRA diagnosis truly sunk in, and I realized that my sense of being "different" was validated. The Defining Event was when I realized that my softball career would be over, when I realized that I may have had physical limitations, and when I realized that, yes, something really WAS wrong. I knew that I wouldn't play softball in college, like I'd daydreamed about. I knew I would likely not even be a part of the high school softball team photo in the yearbook.

At that moment, I stood on the pitcher's mound. I was probably having a great game up until that point, because, well, I'll pat myself on the back: during my hey-day, I was always having a great game. However, I was in pain — a lot of pain. Hospital-worthy pain. Pain that, even to this day, I'd never wish upon anyone. It was somewhat late in the game and my coaches were barking at me and I felt that the world was on my shoulders. I just stood there. I literally just stood there. I couldn't throw another pitch, catch another ball, or run another step. At this point, I had graduated from slow-pitch softball to fast-pitch. My shoulder was absolutely shot and couldn't take it anymore. It felt like someone was stretching my arm out of its socket, then twisting it round and round until it could twist no more. Then lighting it on fire. Then sticking a knife through it. This type of pain radiated through my whole body. While my shoulder was the icing on the crappy store-bought cake, my knee was giving me problems, my ankle hurt, and my heart was shattered into a million itsy bitsy pieces. I felt like the guy on the Operation game board. Any slight touch to any part of my body would result in a painful zing. I could never describe the pain of RA to anyone — it is not something that you "get" unless you get it, which I hope you never do. If I had to try to explain it, it would be like this: flu-like aches all over your whole body, with bad sports injuries in all of your joints. It's like post-surgery pain without the surgery. It's zombie-level tired. Simply put, it's awful, and it was rearing its ugly inflamed head on the softball field that day.

Embarrassingly, I began to cry. I don't know if many people noticed. I felt the hottest, fattest tears just steamrolling down my dirt-streaked, sweaty face. I always acted like a tough girl on the field, and often had an air of cockiness about me when I was in uniform. (It was in stark contrast to the timid and shy little girl I was at school, mind you.) I had the attitude of a champion — and champions didn't cry. Until now. The tears were a result of physical and emotional pain. I was in my happy place, but I wasn't happy. I had to limp off the field, with assistance, and leave the game. I moved like I was made of glass and about to shatter at any second. My world, though, was already shattered. I was probably 12 years old or so. That was The Defining Event.

I quit basketball and eventually tried (multiple times) to return to softball, even signing up for the JV team and then quitting, and then trying my luck at playing on the township team when I was 16 years old. However, my body was just done. I was out. At 16, I hung it up. Retire the jersey; Ashley Boynes is no longer a softball All-Star.

I'd go on to later write essays and publicly speak about the experience, explaining to kids with juvenile arthritis that I'd had to give up a sport that I loved, but that I'd nonetheless still hit a home run in the game of life. I'd pepper my public speaking events with sports metaphors and anecdotes about my softball games, all of which were equal parts true and inspiring and sucky. Sucky is an immature word, it's not a word that an intellectual grown-up should use, but I think that an important part of language is letting go of pretense and letting etymology do its thing. So, yeah, while my sports metaphors and softball anecdotes were all inspiring and true, the whole thing was — and still is — rather sucky.

I can't pretend that juvenile rheumatoid arthritis is awesome. No one wants to be sick, and no kid or teenager wants to be different — the school years, for better or for worse, are often all about "fitting in." It's bad enough to be an outcast because, say, you're a spelling-bee-winning book fair enthusiast with so-called buck-teeth and a weird obsession with Paula Abdul and cowboy boots, but, it is even worse to be labeled an outsider because of a disease or disability beyond your control, especially one that is associated with old ladies.

So, yeah, it is sucky that JRA took away my happy place, the place where I best fit in: the softball field. But, I'm not lying when I say that having to give up sports allowed me to find other areas where I could thrive and flourish: namely, writing and dating boys. (But let's focus on that first part.)

I eventually focused on keeping a journal, joining the school newspaper, and carving out a spot on the yearbook staff, eventually becoming Editor-in-Chief. Before I even graduated high school, I was doing freelance writing jobs, reviewing music for student magazines, and interviewing bands backstage at concerts. By the time I'd graduated high school, I'd completed a Journalistic Layout & Design apprenticeship, and independent study courses in Journalism and Fashion Design at various colleges. I can honestly say, although the diagnosis and lack-of-sports were "sucky," that I don't know that I would have turned towards writing and other interests had I not been practically forced to do so. So while I'm not grateful for pain or sickness, I am grateful that it, in some abstract way, helped me to find my calling. So, I'd say that's a home run in its own right.

(And here's where I'll give a shout-out to the South Fayette Township Panthers & Angels softball teams. I remember our respective hunter green and baby blue softball uniforms like it was yesterday.)

THAT TIME I WAS
A CHEERLEADER ... WITH
ARTHRITIS ... ON A HIT LIST

Luckily, not many people have to deal with a serious illness on top of all of the pressures of normal high school life. Luckily, most people are never on a hit list, and never experience death threats firsthand. Luckily, most teenagers don't end up in court or worrying about restraining orders. Luckily, most teenagers don't take medication that causes them to have permanent blind spots in their eyes.

Unluckily, I experienced every single one of those things during my sophomore year of high school. Step right up, and enjoy the show! Welcome to the circus that is my life.

Now that I'm in my 30s, I can look back and say assuredly that middle school and high school are freakin' hard. It was bad enough for me in the late 90s and early 2000s, before the rise of social media, smartphones, and 24/7 connectedness. It was hard enough for me, even with being a reasonably attractive girl with an unremarkable-yet-fairly-popular position in the school social strata. My God. It was hard. So I can't imagine how hard it is for kids in this day and age, or for people who hit those awkward phases even harder than I did, or who were socially outcast in any way. I can truthfully say to anyone and everyone who is bullied: I'm sorry, and I'm with you. That is not a fun ride to be on, and I sadly still experience it at times, even as an adult.

I imagine that most people have probably, at one point or another, faced bullying, felt like an outsider, or came in contact with some type of animosity. If you haven't, then, congratulations. (And I think you're lying.) The truth is, everyone usually feels insecure or maybe even bullied at some point in his or her lives. For some of us, the experiences are more plentiful or ongoing than they are for others.

When I was in middle school, I discovered my love for fashion. Once I got out of my skater/grunge/Airwalks-and-JNCO-jeans phase, I took a cue from MTV and got myself together. My fashion icons of the time were akin to the likes of Cher from the movie *Clueless*, and Britney Spears (before she went crazy.) I truly adored fashion, cutting photos out of magazines at night and sketching outfits that I would put into a fashion design portfolio. I did fashion projects for art class and enrolled in independent studies in fashion design to fill my free periods at school. Fashion was another one of those interests that helped to fill the softball-shaped hole in my heart.

I put a lot of thought into what I would wear, but not everyone appreciated it. Apparently, makeup and skirts and platform shoes were not widely accepted in a time where most girls my age wore Nike t-shirts with wide-legged jeans or Umbro shorts. I never wavered from who I was, though. I endured proudly getting on the school bus in my

24

new outfits, even as mean girls in the back of the bus taunted me and called me a poser and a whore.

When I decided to try out for cheerleading, it got worse. I had always wanted to be a cheerleader, and when I made the JV squad in 9th and 10th grade, I was absolutely ecstatic. There were a lot of jumps and stunts I couldn't do with my JRA, but, I could handle most of the dances and cheers, and I had an absolute blast at games and pep rallies. I might have been sick on the inside, but on the outside, I looked like a real, live cheerleader!

But, the haters and bullies increased. Once, during a theater arts field trip, some girls threw chewed gum in my hair. I had to sit with it like that through an entire 2-hour musical. A teacher had to help me cut it out with scissors when we stopped for lunch. I cried myself to sleep that night. I also had to contend with rumors of bra-stuffing, drama with boys, and then, the biggie: my health. What I was dealing with healthwise in private was bad enough, but to add the extra adolescent nonsense on top of it was a lot to handle.

I would miss some days of school here and there, and I regularly came in late. I was so sore, stiff, and fatigued in the mornings, but I always did my best to maintain good grades. And I did — I continued to be a member of the gifted program and graduated high school with honors. But the bullying didn't cease. I missed the days of Ashley Beaver Bucktooth Boynes. I now was Ashley Boner, or simply just called a slut, a whore, or a wannabe.

The worst part, though, was when people thought I was lying about my illness, or faking things for sympathy. I would get made fun of if I wore an Air Cast or Ace

Bandage to school. I'd get eye rolls and whispers on days when I had to use crutches. The gossip was never-ending when it came to my tardies and absences. And the limping. Oh, the limping was the worst.

Cheerleading got harder as my medications began to lose effectiveness. I recall having to sit out from gym classes and cheer practice due to my levels of pain and physical difficulties. And I limped. I still loved fashion, though, and I loved cheerleading, too. So I didn't quit cheering, and I didn't quit wearing heels and cute outfits. Yes, this was stupid on my behalf. (A true Sick Idiot era.) My limp was bad enough on its own, and only became more pronounced after cheerleading camp or while teetering on strappy stiletto sandals from Charlotte Russe.

I'll never forget the day that I went to get a Mountain Dew out of the vending machine during cheerleading practice (healthy, I know) and a group of the varsity basketball players — many of whom I considered to be good friends, one of whom I may have had a lifelong crush on — were nearby. They saw me limping down the hall in pain, practically dragging my leg, and were mocking me, imitating my gimpy walk to one another as they tried to suppress hushed laughter. I acted like I didn't notice, but I saw and heard the entire thing, and was deeply hurt by the experience, which has been ingrained in me forever. Before I went back to practice, I stopped by the girls' locker room and cried. I was sad that people saw me as a joke, I was sad that friends were making fun of me, and I was feeling a level of extreme physical pain that most people will never feel in their entire lives. It hurt so badly to be mocked for a disability. And in other instances, it hurt equally to be made fun of for just being myself, wearing what I liked, listening to whatever type of music I liked, dating who I wanted to date, and so on.

My frustrations began to mount, but no one would ever know it. I do not think that I even told my closest friends and family what all I was dealing with at the time. I needed knee surgery and needed to switch medications. My cousin/BFF Jacquie came with me to an eye doctor appointment once, and we had fun playing around in the waiting room. She and I gossiped and joked around while I completed the boring-as-all-get-out hour-long field vision test. Little did I know that it would show damage from a medication I'd been on. I found out that I had Bull's Eye Maculopathy, caused by plaquenil, an anti-malarial drug used to treat rheumatic diseases. Most patients don't get this rare side effect, and in most people it goes away. But, I got it, and it was permanent. Blind spots forever — perfect!

I didn't let it stop me, though. I just switched medications and continued on with my life — my life that another student threatened to end.

I was walking down the hall one day when I heard a boy say that he wanted to kill me. The boy wasn't your typical bully type and didn't fit the stereotype that the media has painted about those who threaten or commit school violence. In fact, he was very attractive, and, oddly enough, I'd always liked him, and found him to be much cooler and more interesting than other boys our age. I wasn't sure where the animosity came from, although I knew he made fun of the types of trendy clothes that I wore and the Top 40 pop music that I listened to. So, although hearing this hurt my feelings, I ignored his comment. I did tell a friend about it, though, rolling my eyes and casually brushing it off. Apparently, a concerned teacher and another student overheard this exchange nonetheless, and told the principal.

That night, I was out at a fancy dinner for my good friend Valerie's birthday. We were with a large group at a lovely restaurant atop Mt. Washington, overlooking the gorgeous night skyline of Pittsburgh when my little pink flip phone rang. Let me be clear that, at this time, cell phones were not used the way they are today. If someone was calling me, it was important. It was my mom calling.

"Did something happen at school today that you would like to tell me about?" she asked.

I felt knots in my stomach. I was a teenager. I'm sure a lot happened that day, and I'm sure that I wanted to tell her zero of it.

"No?" I answered, tentatively. It came out like a question.

She proceeded to tell me that the school called because a student threatened my life. He was expelled, they were searching his locker, police were involved — it was a big ordeal.

It turned out that three of the other girls at the dinner that night, along with myself, a male friend of ours, and a teacher, were on a hit list. Now, this was after the Columbine school shootings but way before the other terrible acts of school violence that sadly seem to be the norm today, and so I guess that the school probably handled the situation okay, given the circumstances.

But talk about drama! We had to go to court, there was a restraining order involved, we had to speak in front of the school board, and so on. Apparently they found enough "evidence" in his locker and on his website that was cause for concern. At the time, I worried about his welfare, believe it or not. I didn't want to incriminate this kid who I had respected, and who was once my friend. Besides, no high school student wants to be a tattletale or a snitch. The whole thing was a nightmare for all involved.

I still don't harbor any ill feelings towards him, but am flabbergasted now, as an adult, about how blasé I was about the whole thing back then. My friends and I thought the entire situation was absurd, and it seemed like we thought it was a not as big a deal as it was. We'd tended to kind of laugh it off, as teenagers do. I now see naïve that was, though, given the acts of violence that teenagers have committed in schools since then. I don't believe that he was a true threat, but who knows. Reflecting on the "what could have been," as an adult, is terrifying. I think that, understandably, it was around this time when I first developed some veiled anxiety.

I eventually had to quit cheerleading. The jumps and gymnastics skills that were required were not something I was remotely able to do. So, I hung up the pom-poms along with that ol' softball jersey. People continued to make fun of my limp, and sometimes my clothes, but never again was I on a hit list that I know of.

That was high school, for ya. There were a lot of wonderful memories, too, of course, and sometimes I wish that I could go back — but it certainly wasn't without its share of ups and downs. After all was said and done, during my senior year I won Most Stylish, Most Crush-worthy, and Most Likely to be Famous. We could only pick one senior superlative, though, and so I chose Most Stylish, as a not-so-subtle middle finger to those back-of-the-bus bullies who made fun of the way I dressed for all those years. (Plus, Biggest Sick Idiot wasn't a category. I would have won that one unanimously.)

THAT TIME MY FACE WAS PARALYZED AND I GOT MY OWN PUPPY

College is a time of growth, independence, and self-discovery. It's a time for new friends, new experiences, and, sometimes, new love. It is a time where many will — literally and figuratively — stumble along their path to true adulthood. I know that I, for one, stumbled a few times, in both senses.

I also learned a lot about my character and the character of others during this chaotic period of my life when I was grasping at straws not only figuring out who I was as a young woman, but also trying to figure out my health.

I was constantly tired — more tired than a typical 20-something should have been. Even with a full course load, a bustling social life, a steady boyfriend, a part time job, multiple internships, and various student organizations, I was still too exhausted for it to be considered even remotely normal. I was constantly ill: brain fog, sore throats, swollen glands, and headaches, on top of my joint pain and stiffness from rheumatoid arthritis.

I somehow made it through the fall semester of my sophomore year at Clarion University of Pennsylvania without incident. But then, when I was visiting home one weekend early on in the spring semester, I felt even more fatigued than usual, and knew that something was off. My boyfriend at the time (now ex) was hanging out with me at my parents' house. We watched a movie — *Reservoir Dogs*, if my memory serves me correctly — until he had to leave. When he kissed me goodbye, I noticed that I couldn't feel it on the left side of my face or mouth.

"Do I look funny?" I asked.

"Do you want me to answer that?" he joked in reply.

"No, seriously," I insisted.

He stared at me.

"No, you look fine," he answered.

I explained that my face felt numb, which we agreed was strange, but not necessarily cause for concern. I'd often experienced the most random of symptoms, and so it didn't seem implausible that this was a side effect from a medication or, what I like to refer to as, a "me-issue."

See, in my mind, there's "me-sick" and "normal-person-sick." This is how I try to objectively gauge what is going on with my health at any given time: is it cause for concern for me? Would it be a cause of concern for a normal person? Is it just a symptom that is "normal" for my chronic health issues and me? Or, am I normal-person sick i.e. dealing with some kind of acute illness unrelated to any of my chronic conditions?

Up until this point, my facial weirdness seemed to be an isolated "me-issue" that I needn't worry about. It seemed to be a sporadic event that was related to my general chronic health problems and not necessarily something new or that needed to be a cause for concern. It didn't feel like an emergency.

About an hour or so after Ex-Boyfriend left, my younger brother came home after a night out with friends. By this point, I was fairly certain something was wrong, but I was too tired and too invested in an episode of *the Real World* to be bothered to get up and go look in a mirror. (Again, as hindsight would have it, not my best life decision. Classic Sick Idiot.)

"Oh my God. Ash. You need to go to the hospital," my brother Ryan said when he saw me.

He had a friend with him who started wigging out when he saw me, later stating that it "looked like my face was melting off."

This, naturally, is not something you ever want to hear, and it freaked me out. We woke my parents, and the decision was made that if it wasn't better by morning, we'd see my doctor first thing. (After all, it could have just been a "me-issue" that would be gone as quickly as it'd come about, and it seemed that I was making a mountain out of a molehill. I can become a bit fixated when it comes to my appearance.)

By the next morning it had gotten noticeably worse. We called and promptly headed to the doctor. Ah, let me tell you about this particular doctor — quite a gem, this one.

He wasn't a specialist, just a general family doctor. He wasn't good for much more than a yearly physical and calling in an antibiotic here and there. To avoid being sued, I won't say too much more. But, I need to preface this all by stating that this guy thought I was a hypochondriac.

Now, let me be clear: I'm not. I WISH I were. If I were, that would mean that I wasn't sick, at least not physically sick, which would be pretty awesome. If I were able to erase the physical misery that I live with more frequently than not, I would. I really wish that I were simply making things up for attention, that I was simply drug-seeking, that I was crazy, that this book and the stories contained within it were fiction. Those things would all probably make more sense than the multitude of crazy health situations I've been in over these first three decades of my life. I wish that I were imaginative enough to come up with half of the things I've dealt with … but, no, I'm not a hypochondriac. As they say, truth is stranger than fiction, and so is my health history.

So, anyway, the next morning, we go to this lovely doctor, who ever-so-graciously squeezed me in for an appointment. It took a couple of calls and some pleading. I mean, after all, what's the urgency of a 21-year-old who looks like she had a stroke? We got there and found that he was, as per usual, clueless. He smiled a lot and it annoyed me. In my head I called him Dr. McDummy, which says a mouthful. My mom basically had to tell him that I needed to go to the ER and that we only came to him to get a prescription for an MRI, stat. She had to suggest the possibility of Bell's Palsy to him while he scratched his head and probably daydreamed about

Teletubbies or *Hannah Montana*. She may have even given him a sticker or a lollipop while he made some calls on a big boy phone and jotted some notes down like a real live grown-up. I do not recall, but, before we set off to the hospital, he probably wrote me a crayon-penned prescription for an antibiotic, and told me that it was all in my head ... because that was all he ever did.

(As you can tell, I have a lot of respect for this guy — approximately as much respect as he had for me through the years. And I'm only mildly overstating his elementary level of proficiency.)

We spent the day at the hospital. I do remember MRIs and blood work, perhaps a CT scan and x-ray, too. I don't remember many details. I'm not sure if I was highly drugged up at this point, or, if I was just experiencing a heavy kind of brain fog due to my lovely new condition. Ex-Boyfriend came to sit with my mom while I'd had the tests done. He seemed genuinely worried, and that was one of the last actual nice things I remember him doing. (The stories from that relationship could be an entire book in and of themselves, but since I actually respect him more than Dr. McDummy, I won't say too much more about him, other than I appreciate his being there for me during this time when I felt grotesque, even if he did cheat on me and throw my health issues in my lopsided face on occasion, claiming me that he, "stayed with me when I looked like a f**king special ed student." NOT COOL ON ANY LEVEL, IN ANY UNIVERSE.)

I would eventually be diagnosed with a condition called Bell's Palsy. Doctors do not know what causes it, though it is suspected to perhaps stem from a virus. One of my more difficult college memories was having to take a medical withdrawal for the semester, pack up my dorm room (with the help of two friends to whom I will be ever-grateful) and make the 2-hour ride back home with my parents. I would be on bed rest, taking a high dose of steroids, and would gain 35-lbs to hit my highest-ever weight during the following three months.

I should probably take this opportunity to explain to you all that I'm admittedly a little on the vain side. Okay, maybe a lot on the vain side. I am not shallow, by any means. There is a difference. I do care about far more than my looks. I know true beauty comes from within, and I'm completely comfortable in sweats, glasses, and a makeup-free face. But that said, I can nonetheless be a tad vain. I own up to my vanity, and the people in my life have come to accept it. However, "accept it" was something that I could not do during this time. I felt fat, sick, and hideous. My eye and my mouth drooped down and my entire face was literally lopsided. I was puffy from steroids, and I had never weighed so much or felt so ugly in my entire life. Bell's Palsy ruined my self-esteem, and I barely wanted to leave my house. It was perhaps a good thing, though, because I wasn't feeling well enough to leave my house, anyway. My face may have been paralyzed, but the accompanying fatigue was also paralyzing. I felt like all I did was sleep, and it became somewhat of a boring and lonely existence.

A favorite memory of mine during this time of me living as a hermit was something so utterly simple. I'd been having a rough time, and my grandparents picked me up from my parents' house where I was living at the time, and took me to Barnes & Noble to pick out some books and enjoy a chai from Starbucks. I remember that one of the books I'd gotten was a journal, and I thus began to write again. I consider this to be part of the silver lining of an all-around ugly situation.

The other silver lining was the little blessing who came my way, named LucyLoo. I had wanted a puppy forever, and at this time was pretty set on a yorkie or a pug. My family had an Airedale Terrier named Dezzie who I adored, but I wanted my own little dog, too. Perhaps it was out of pity, but my mom and dad caved and allowed me to start the hunt for a new pup. It took a while, but we finally found an ad for pug mixes that needed a home. My Mom and I drove to West Virginia, not sure what we would encounter.

What we found was a box full of what looked to be purebred pugs, and one scrawny, somewhat sickly-looking pup with lighter, longer, and more wiry hair. She was almost silver in color, and was teeny-tiny and frail, albeit, adorable. The little pipsqueak kept running up to me, and I would pick her up, but my mom was unsure because she didn't look as healthy or as "puggy" as the others. Nonetheless, my heart melted for her. When her misfit self ran up to me one last time and smothered my lopsided face with kisses, I knew that she had chosen me, and that we were meant to be. Our hearts simply belonged together. I couldn't reject her for looking sickly – after all, I did, too.

We both were misfits in our own rights, with silly-looking faces that were seemingly meant to lay eyes upon one another at that time.

I named her LucyLoo, and we were inseparable from that moment on. I ended up thanking God for my Bell's Palsy in a way, because, without it, I may have not rediscovered my love for writing, and I may not have found, as Edith Wharton once said, "my little dog … my heartbeat at my feet."

THAT TIME I WAS NAMED CRASHLEY AND GOT REAR-ENDED ON NEW YEAR'S EVE

Let's make something clear from the get-go. Driving and I haven't mixed too well over the years. In fact, it earned me yet another nickname: Crashley. (Though, I prefer my family's lifelong nickname for me, Buella.) I used to be very sensitive about my driving record, but now I laugh it off. I've gotten better and as they say, you live, you learn. During high-school, I had a few incidents: running into the garage wall, being hit by a deer, hitting a deer, rear-ending someone, and an unfortunate merging incident that actually wasn't my fault. Then, there were times my car broke down on the highway, or in the snow, or at school. Thank goodness for friends with jumper cables (Glenn!) and my amazing dad who can fix anything and everything — including a plethora of my sometimes-totaled cars. (Without him, I would have been that person who is always mooching a ride. No one wants to be that person.)

Understandably, though, driving started to "activate" a bit of that anxiety that I'd referenced earlier. While being on a hit list and dealing with medical issues may have started it off, being Crashley didn't help the cause. My first full-blown panic attack was when I was driving to college. Through the years, I'd have many a panic attack while driving or while stuck in traffic. To this day, even though my anxiety is pretty under control, driving (and flying — I love traveling, but hate traveling in airplanes) is a trigger.

You'd think with this kind of mentality that I'd be more careful and responsible than I was — even overly so. I got a few speeding tickets, a lot of parking tickets, and had a reckless driving incident. My ex-boyfriends didn't help my vehicular anxiety. Without getting too far into it, I'll say that maliciously and irresponsibly speeding around in a vehicle with your girlfriend in the passenger seat — just to scare her — is a form of mental abuse, in my humble opinion. I had not one, but two, ex-boyfriends do this to me, over petty stuff. (One, because he felt like it, was jealous over an outfit I'd worn to school, and was amped up by an Eminem song. The other, because he was an unpredictable asshole, who had possessed more than a smattering of crazy.)

I eventually became a responsible driver/vehicle owner, and eventually was no longer dating those jerks or having panic attacks when I would drive through the many tunnels of my fair city. To celebrate my newfound independence (I was single! My RA was under control! My Bell's Palsy was gone! I transferred to my beloved University of Pittsburgh!) I decided to start the new year off right. I dressed myself in a lacy black top with blank pants and black heels. My hair? Wild and curly. My attitude? Beyoncé. My cleavage? On display. And, before I went, I injected myself with my latest biologic drug, Enbrel, because what could be sexier on New Year's Eve than a girl with arthritis? *Boo-ya!*

Anyway, after I took <u>that</u> shot, I headed out to celebrate with friends in the South Side of Pittsburgh, with the hopes of taking a more fun kind of shot. (Flaming Dr. Pepper? Washington Apple? Lemon Drops? Jägerbombs? The possibilities were endless.) The plan was to drive to my friend's apartment, where I would park my vehicle. We would then walk (or limp, depending on how my old-lady knee held up in heels,) to our various locales for the evening, and I would be a responsible adult and stay the night at said apartment. It was a plan that could not be foiled! Crashley would not come out to play.

"Be careful, watch out for deer!" my dad told me as I left the house.

But, as my luck would have it, I got rear-ended (hard!) by a guy going 40 MPH, while I was at a complete stop. It wasn't pretty, and to this day, I still have neck issues that, coupled with some underlying health conditions, could very likely have been triggered by this lovely incident on that fateful evening. So what does a young 20-something who is dressed to the nines, all dolled up for a night of fun, do in this situation? I did exchange insurance and contact information with the driver. I certainly didn't call the police or an ambulance. I also surely did not tell anyone that my neck hurt — after all, no one wants to share a New Year's Eve kiss with a Sick Idiot, *amiright?*

Perhaps that was one of those "hindsight-is-20-20" issues and perhaps I should have sought out medical treatment for my neck but, *meh*. Your twenties are for mistakes and random road trips and New Year's Eve parties. I may not have gotten a kiss at midnight that year … but my year, unfortunately, did start out with a bang that I, and my neck, will always remember.

THAT TIME I MET MY FUTURE HUSBAND AND MY BEST FRIEND WAS IN A COMA

I have kissed a lot of frogs, and none of them turned into Prince Charming. I began dating at the age of 15, and by my mid-20s, was wondering if a knight-in-shining armor was ever going to show up to complete my Sick Idiot fairy tale. While I'm mixing metaphors here, let's just say: there are a lot of fish in the sea, and it felt like I dated most of them. Unfortunately, the majority of these guys were less like fish, and more like the Loch Ness Monster.

I am not one to hold grudges, so I won't give away too many specifics or call anyone out by name, but to be clear, I have dealt with some crap. Sure, there were some good things: thoughtful gifts, poems and love notes, being serenaded by guitar, talks of the future, date nights, and romance. Some of these experiences and these relationships helped to shape me into who I am today. But there were the not-so-great-moments, too.

I had one boyfriend who was emotionally unstable and mentally abusive, and who liked to throw things, including both temper tantrums and physical objects. He is also the Ex-Boyfriend mentioned earlier who made fun of my

Bell's Palsy after the fact, told me I looked "stupid" when I limped, and yelled expletives at my parents about me at two o'clock in the morning.

I had my high school sweetheart cheat on me the night of his graduation. I had one guy break up with me in a text message, like the modern-day equivalent of the Sex & the City episode where Carrie gets dumped via Post-It. (This was the only time I'd ever been broken up with, instead of vice versa, and it was via text message. Go figure.) I had the crazy-driving lads mentioned in the previous chapter, and I've had one boyfriend just leave me at a bar. One of my exes was an Eminem song personified. One spread rumors about me to some NFL players (long story.) One guy had religious beliefs that I couldn't agree with. He was nice, sweet, and talented, but he also talked about his poop at Thanksgiving. I've had the guys who told me they loved me when it was simply way too late. I've had the ones who have cheated, multiple times — and I was gullible enough to take them back. I dated one guy who offered to pay off a $300 credit card balance for me, and then, when we broke up, sent an email to my parents demanding they repay him. These were some gems. I dealt with jealousy, possessiveness, and general psychotic behavior.

I didn't realize it at the time, but I put up with a lot of nonsense that I truly didn't deserve. You see, I was a serial monogamist. By the time I graduated from college, I had been in three relationships that had lasted 2-3 years a piece — pretty serious for someone my age. I was not typically single for long, and when I entered into a relationship, I stuck with it until I could not do so any longer. I just loved love. I never was one to need a man, but I simply liked being with somebody. That said, I could have used more discernment with who those somebodies were. I needed less Loch Ness Monsters in my life. In hindsight, if I were to psychoanalyze myself, I'd say that my being sick caused me to view myself as damaged goods, which maybe caused me to feel like being treated as such was okay. Having a physical disability or health problem can bring a lot of baggage to any relationship, friendship, or professional partnership. As my health issues grew worse through college, I think that my self-esteem went downhill.

Then, something shifted. I decided to just focus on me. I dated around and met some nice people. I just enjoyed my life for a little bit. I went out and made fun memories with my girlfriends. (One Halloween, I even saved my friend Eileen's life by limping to a pay phone in a bumblebee costume while her apartment was on fire, but that's a whole other story for a whole other book.) I focused on myself, on having fun, and on cultivating friendships. While finally focusing on loving my life instead of living for a guy, a good guy came along after what seemed like an eternity of games and heartbreak, with some unrequited love and major melodrama thrown in for good measure.

I'll spare you all the story of our courtship and our romance, because I think that some things should be kept relatively private. But, suffice it to say, I knew early on that Mike was special. In fact, I felt so comfortable with him on our first date that I told him about my rheumatoid arthritis nearly immediately. It was not exactly your typical first-date topic of conversation, but I figured that he might as well know about it up front. The greatest part of doing so right off the bat was that I found out that it somehow didn't matter to him.

He has been by my side ever since. Through diagnosis after diagnosis, seeing me at both my best and my worst, Mike has truly been there through sickness and through health — and he married me knowing full well what he was getting into. I'm sure that the extent of it has, at times, surprised him — I know that my health consistently continues to surprise even me — but he's been there. It felt good to know that he saw enough good in me to outweigh the negative baggage, and was attracted enough to me to overlook my health problems. He saw me as more than damaged goods.

I knew fairly early on that he would be a rock for me when I needed it most. The summer after we began dating, one of my best friends, Nicole, was in a bad accident that left her in a coma. We didn't know what her fate would be. I visited her at the hospital almost every day on my lunch break, and would cry to Mike about it at night. He would reassure me that everything would be okay, and after a long road, because Nicole is a strong woman and a survivor, it was. His presence during that time when I was consumed with sadness and worry for my friend was crucial.

Nicole's accident also made me realize how fragile life is. It reminded me that every day is a gift. It made me appreciate the good in life instead of focusing on my problems at the time, which were comparatively smaller. Her long road to finding her new normal has continually inspired me. She has persevered on, through ups and downs, and we now are able to share with one another when it comes to dealing with health woes and pain.

As for my exes, I truly wish them all nothing but the best. I can say that, if nothing else, they taught me that I could overcome heartbreak in addition to any other condition that life would throw at me. They also taught me, that some people live with pain, while some people live with pains in the asses. I'm just glad that I'm not doing the latter anymore.

THAT TIME I GOT CARRIED OUT OF A CATHEDRAL

During college, I savored reading the classics. I took a particular liking to the Victorian era of British literature, and women's literature. I also dug Nicholas Sparks, because, duh.

However, my love for the written word did not stop there. I took as many English electives as I could, which wasn't hard considering my concentrations in English Literature, English Writing, and Communications. I took Children's Literature (loved it!), a class on Shakespeare (loved it!), Bible as Literature (hated it!) and one (very boring) American Lit class which was so unremarkable that I could not tell you anything we read besides *Robinson Crusoe*. In case you're wondering why this specific book stands out in my card catalog of literati memories, it isn't because I particularly liked the story, or because my professor taught it in an interesting or thought-provoking manner. It stands out because the professor seemed to be utterly obsessed with Robinson Crusoe and "his boy, Friday." If there were a fan club for these two characters, this stodgy ol' prof would have been fanboy #1.

I don't recall his name, sadly, but we'll just call him The Crusoe Fanboy. One spring day, as The Crusoe Fanboy rambled on, and on, and on, and I fought the urge to take an afternoon snooze, I noticed an uncomfortable sensation. No, it wasn't his incessant droning making me cringe with every syllable, though that was part of it. It wasn't the scalding hot peppermint tea that I'd burnt my tongue on as I hurried to class. (I was always late.)

It was my knee.

Before I continue, I'll set the stage by saying that after a couple of transfers and a medical leave, I finally attended the (awesome) University of Pittsburgh, whose crown jewel, in my opinion, is the gorgeous Cathedral of Learning. The gothic revival architecture is worth a tour or a least a photo-op if you're ever sightseeing in Pittsburgh. The history contained within its walls is something to be respected, and I always felt a little bit like a student of Hogwarts as I roamed the dark hallways, admiring the beauty of the building with every rushed journey to my next class.

The reason I mention the Cathedral is because it is important to note that it is pretty old, and has some questionable design features that likely weren't really of much concern when it was built in 1926. For example, despite there being some wheelchair ramps, there was not an elevator anywhere near my classroom, only steps. These steps and my knee didn't always get along.

At any rate, on this fateful day, my knee started feeling … weird. It wasn't necessarily hurting; I wasn't in excruciating pain. But it was an uncomfortable sensation that I had never felt before. Now, my knee had given me problems plenty of times up until that point — my knee issues weren't news to me. It was one of my first joints "to go," as they say, and is luckily one of the only joints of mine that suffered any kind of permanent irreversible damage or destruction. It's a disaster in there — bone on bone, no joint space, some bone spurs and calcium deposits, a piece of meniscus floating around, and so on. Between a skiing injury, rheumatoid arthritis, years of sports (including cheerleading which, yes, is a sport,) and the onset of osteoarthritis, I had one doctor tell me that he was surprised I could walk, so that's pretty telling. I had my first arthroscopic surgery around 1998, and my second in 2010. The great irony of this is that I was told when I was 25 years old that I could certainly use a total knee replacement ... but that I was too young, and most surgeons would advise against it. So on paper, I'm a great candidate, but in practice, I'm not.

The Great Cathedral of Learning/Crusoe Fanboy incident of 2007(ish) was even before my second scope surgery, though — a surgery that, apparently, I should have gotten done sooner than I did. As I was sitting in that ever-so-stimulating borefest of a class, I suddenly realized that I was completely, utterly, screwed. My knee that started off as being simply "uncomfortable" was now locked in a 90-degree angle. I panicked a little bit. It was not simply "stiff" — a stretch would not do. I literally could not move it. It was mechanically, physically, seemingly-permanently stuck in that position, and there was absolutely no way that it was unbending any time soon.

I did what any image-conscious early-twentysomething would do — and that was NOT DRAW ANY NEGATIVE ATTENTION TO MYSELF. I did not want these classmates who I barely knew knowing my true secret identity as Sick Idiot. All most of them knew of me is that 1.) I was consistently late, 2.) I usually had a Starbucks drink in my hand, and 3.) I was a suck-up. (I may not have liked the class, the reading material, or the professor, but I liked knowing the right answers in class and sharing my wealth of knowledge. You're welcome, classmates!)

It wasn't the type of course structure that facilitated student conversations or group interactions, and Pitt was a large campus. No one in my social circle was in the class with me, and, in that moment, I regretted not having an in-class friend to pass a note to for some kind of help or advice. So, I would have to wait it out for a full 90-minutes — one for each degree in which my leg was bent. I tried to blend in, to not look like I was panicking and hurting. (Yeah, at some point "uncomfortable" turns to "painful" when your knee is stuck like that.)

As I continued to try not to be noticed, I tried to also slyly pull out my cell phone, which was strictly prohibited. I couldn't let The Crusoe Fanboy see me, or I really would be drawing attention to myself, not to mention, I'd be in trouble. So, I kept it on the down low and tried to text my boyfriend (now husband) who was out of college and working a grown-up job as a schoolteacher. Well, aside from not-always-accessible elevators, another awesome part of the Cathedral of Learning at that time was that cellular service was spotty, at best. So, many unsuccessful texting attempts later, I resigned to my fate of being forever stuck in the most boring classroom on earth.

When The Crusoe Fanboy finished his lengthy monologue on the awesomeness of his homies RC and BF, the other students began gathering up their belongings, and slowly filing out of the classroom to enjoy the lovely spring day. I slowly packed away my notebook, planner, pen, cell phone, lip balm, and highlighter. I realized that I still had to stall. I didn't want my classmates witnessing the sure atrocity that would be my attempt at standing up on my own. I tried to make it look like I was searching for something in a folder while the last of the stragglers made their way out of the room. I'm sure I got some odd glances as I sat there awkwardly, especially considering that I was typically the first one to book it out the door the second I had the chance.

Finally, it was only myself and The Crusoe Fanboy left. Calling him Fanboy is funny, because he was probably nearing the age of 80 and could hardly qualify as a "boy." I doubted that his frail, wrinkly old frame would do me much good in this situation. He certainly wasn't going to be able to carry me out of the classroom, and I didn't know if he'd be willing to put down his copy of *Robinson Crusoe* long enough to even be able to do so.

I stifled a laugh at the picture of this grumpy old professor somehow hoisting me over his shoulders like a strapping young lad. Superman, he was not. He stared at me uncomfortably the question of "what the hell I was doing there" lingering in the air.

"Did you need something?" he asked.

It was the first time he'd ever spoken to me, and maybe any other human being, outside of teaching. I turned beet red. I had no idea how I'd explain myself, because, let's be honest — how do you explain something so absurd? So, I did what I do best: I rambled.

Over-explaining, I countered,

"Um, well, I have arthritis. The autoimmune kind. I've had juvenile rheumatoid arthritis since I was 10. Well, my knee is one of my bad joints. I don't know what happened, but as I was sitting here, it locked up. Like, completely froze. It's stuck. Literally. I don't need to stretch, it isn't stiff, it's really just stuck. Like, mechanically stuck. I can't move it."

He looked at me with a mixture of discomfort, confusion, pity, and concern.

"Oh, okay. Take your time," was his reply, as he grabbed his trench coat and briefcase. At a loss for words, I stared at him, with my mouth gaping. Was he really just going to leave me there?

"What can I do for you?" he finally asked. I sense that he was suppressing a sigh or an eye-roll, but I can't be sure.

"Uhh, I don't know. I mean, I'm trying to call my boyfriend to come get me. I can't walk to my car, it's parked really far away today. I don't know how I'm getting out of the building or even getting downstairs," I explained. If I recall correctly, I was on the 6th floor or so. The whole "steps" thing wasn't going to work out for me if I was riding solo throughout this debacle.

"Maybe you can just help me get up out of my chair and out into the hallway so I can see if I have cell service there and figure out what to do?" I asked with trepidation.

"Okay," he said. I thought I saw an inkling of compassion gleam across his face, but I still sensed that he was harboring some annoyance or exasperation.

I hoisted my purse and my tote onto my shoulder and tried to stand up with the assistance of his arm, the desk, and my one good leg.

"Can you put your foot down at all?" he asked me.

I glanced at him blankly. Hadn't he heard me explain that I literally couldn't move my knee at all? He, of all people, should know that an English major would not use the word literally unless she meant it literally!

"No, I can't," I said. "I can try to hop."

So with his assistance, I hopped my way up to the front of the classroom, silently bemoaning my propensity towards always sitting at the back of the class. The hopping seemed appropriate, as this was my last class before Easter break. I wondered if the Easter Bunny felt as stupid hopping around as I did.

Luckily, there was a bench in the hall right outside the classroom where I could sit and rest and wait for some kind of rescue, be it Mike, Superman, or SpongeBob Square Pants — I really didn't care, I just needed help. Unluckily, there was not an elevator that was within hopping distance — at least not for a hopping amateur like myself. The Easter Bunny may have been able to hop that far, but not this girl.

"Will you be okay?" The Crusoe Fanboy asked, with a look that was barely disguising his urge to flee the scene. I didn't know the answer to that question, but I owed the man some kind of reply.

"Yeah, I'll be okay. This is embarrassing. Thank you so much for your help! Really, thank you! Have a nice Easter," I gushed.

He rushed off and the incident, which was incredibly awkward for us both, was never again mentioned, neither by me nor by The Crusoe Fanboy. (Though, I think it's important to mention that I was truly grateful for his assistance … just not quite as grateful for his in-class lectures.)

I tried my phone again. I had one little meager bar of service — a bar that, at that time, looked like my lifeline. I repeatedly took turns calling my parents and my boyfriend and a few of my friends until finally Mike picked up. I explained my situation and then had to wait a grueling half hour or so until he was able to get to me.

This was the first time since we'd been dating that he'd actually seen me as full-on Sick Idiot. He'd heard legendary tales of Sick Idiot, he'd perhaps seen photographic evidence of Sick Idiot, but he had never had the full Sick Idiot Experience live and in-person. I didn't know if it was more humiliating that I, as a young college girl, had to be helped out of a classroom by an elderly man — who was my teacher, for God's sake! — or, that my hot new boyfriend had to see me in Sick Idiot mode.

When he arrived, we had to deduce how the hell we'd get me out of the Cathedral. He would either have to carry me down the steps (thank goodness he's a fitness fanatic,) or he'd have to carry me to the way-out-of-the-way elevator. So, he carried me down approximately 6 flights of stairs. It sounds super-romantic, like a real Disney princess/damsel-in-distress moment, but it was super embarrassing for me.

Once we got outside, I decided I'd try my hand at being a hop-along. I really didn't want my peers seeing me being carried around the campus. Somehow, me standing on at least one of my own two legs seemed to be slightly more dignified, gimpy as it was. And so that's what we did. I leaned on him, he grabbed on to me, and as I fended off many a strange look, I hopped my way (many blocks, in a pretty bustling metropolitan area) to his car, as we figured out a way for my parents to come and pick up mine.

At some point on the way home, as luck would have it, my knee unlocked. Of course, it couldn't have been as cooperative during class, whilst leaning on my old-man professor, or while humiliating myself in front of my boyfriend and entire college campus, but at least it unlocked itself on its own time. (However, that wouldn't be the last time that my knee would lock up, unfortunately.)

We took a ride to a chiropractor who was able to loosen it up a little more. One thing he couldn't put back into place, though, was my ego, which was bruised, broken, and left behind me somewhere on the 6th floor of the Cathedral of Learning.

THAT TIME I HAD A BEEF WITH GLUTEN AND A NUN

After earning my Bachelor's Degree, I was uncertain as to what my career path would be. I got a good job with a startup social media app as a marketing coordinator, but unfortunately due to budget issues, was laid off along with half of the marketing team after a short period of time. I'd take other jobs here and there, including one at the eBay consignment website that I'd worked for alongside my younger brother Ryan during college. Interestingly enough, while I was at that company, I came close to getting shot when a co-worker accidentally shot a gun in the cubicle next to me. He was inspecting and researching the antiquated weapon as part of our intake and examination process when it inadvertently fired. Thank God, who will probably be disappointed in me after this chapter, that it was not loaded. I'm telling you — my life is stranger than fiction. To this day, I have pretty prominent tinnitus (ringing in my ears,) and I wonder if this could be part of the cause. (This, and vitamin deficiencies, and always wanting front-row seats to loud concerts.)

Anyway, though I loved this company, it was clear that it wasn't going to be my full-time "forever" job. I knew I wanted to be a writer, but, at the time, I didn't know how to translate that into a career. My health issues were fairly under control thanks to Enbrel, and, more out of uncertainty than anything else, I toyed around with the idea of going back to school for education. I thought I wanted the routine stability that I felt it would offer. A lot of my friends were teachers, my boyfriend was a teacher, and the thought of teaching English definitely appealed to me on some level.

So since I didn't know what else to do, I applied and was accepted into grad school. In just two years, I'd have my Master's Degree in Education from the Indiana University of Pennsylvania. My first year would be coursework, and the second would be an immersion/student-teaching experience. In Pennsylvania, teaching is an extremely difficult field to get into. We have some of the best school districts in the country, and the teachers in Pennsylvania are relatively well-paid in comparison to the rest of the United States. So, during my time in graduate school, I figured I needed some kind of edge. While my portfolio was shaping up to be pretty impressive, and I was getting great grades in my courses, I knew that I had to get a teaching-related job, and fast.

I searched high and low, and found some small gigs. I tutored a Korean graduate student in English as a Second Language. I worked at an elementary after-school program at a small private academy. It was great, but I wasn't sure that it was enough. I finally took the plunge and started emailing some smaller Catholic schools in the area to see if they needed substitute teachers, tutors, or coaches.

As luck (whether good or bad luck remains to be seen) would have it, the Catholic church that I attended had a small elementary and middle school, and they were in need of a school secretary. I applied and was hired by a charming gray-haired nun. I was so excited. I bought all of the cutesy, teacherly stuff to jazz up my desk and my work area. I loved my thematic and seasonally-appropriate Miss Boynes banners and the fun magnets on my filing cabinet. I loved seeing the kids each morning, and I became friends with many of the teachers and some of the children's parents. It became a nice, routine little job, and I was able to leave work early enough to make it to my evening graduate classes.

Of course, my body had to adjust to getting up so early, to being cooped up indoors all day, and to the stress of handling a full-time job and full-time master's-level coursework all at once. For a normal person, it would be challenging. For a person living in a constant state of inflammation and autoimmunity, it was nearly nightmarish. My body did not adjust well. The Sick Idiot started to show her ugly face. It started off by coming in late here and there. Then, it moved to vomiting in the bathroom almost every morning. I had morning sickness without being pregnant. Migraines were triggered by the musty, stifling smell of the school office. One time, the lunch lady thought I was having a seizure. On several occasions I nearly passed out. Simply put, I was going downhill and not doing so hot.

I was barely able to focus, but I did the work that needed to be done each day. The things that were important were handled. Attendance was taken, lunches were ordered, mail was in the teacher's mailboxes, and copies were made. Believe it or not, I was seriously also the school nurse, despite zero official medical training: ta-da!

I even volunteered to be the cheerleading coach, and to sub as a teacher as-needed, on top of my full-time school secretary job (which, ask any school secretary, is a daunting career choice that is not for the faint of heart.) There was some busywork that would fall to the wayside, particularly if I was battling a migraine, or vomiting, or having an RA flare in my fingers. An example of said busywork would be retyping decades-old registration files on a typewriter — and for no apparent reason. But, I did my best. The teachers who I worked with were compassionate and empathetic. They didn't get to interact with me much during the day, but they knew I was struggling and were very kindhearted about it. (Fun fact? One of the preschool teachers was the mother of the kid who almost shot me at the eBay place. How's that for full circle?)

My boss at the time was the school principal, a.k.a. the now-not-as-charming gray-haired nun. Now, you may think that I am automatically going to Hell for talking poorly about a nun, but, as you continue reading, you will understand. I've got to vent about this. I will repent later. If she reads this, I ask her (and God) for forgiveness in advance.

I have to start off by saying that she was completely sweet-old-lady-charming when she wanted to be, but she also smelled. So did the school office. The office itself had a musty, moldy odor … but the nun … man, she just smelled. I feel so mean for even mentioning it, but it was to the point that it was offensive. I know she had a lot on her plate, and a very stressful job — I mean, what could be more stressful than God being your boss? But it seemed as though she never took the time to partake in personal grooming or hygiene habits. If odors weren't one of my primary migraine triggers, it wouldn't have bothered me as much. But the smells of her and the office combined were absolutely suffocating.

That said, I wouldn't even broach the topic of her stench if she didn't also stink as a person sometimes on top of it. She obviously is, on some level, a good person, if she devoted her life to the church. I can respect that, I give her credit for that, and I honor her for it. There were glimpses of kindness, when she allowed me to come in a little later in the morning than originally agreed upon, when she struggled to make some special accommodations for me, when she would occasionally take my suggestions for the school newsletter, and when she got me a nice Christmas present during the holidays and sent me flowers once when I was sick. She was sweet to most of the kids, and was an utter doll when the priests were around.

But…

Whether intentional or not, she was so downright, bitterly nasty to me sometimes that it was absolutely ridiculous. Other people noticed it, too. See, I have this odd pattern of getting stuck with horrible bosses … like, I could have starred in the *Horrible Bosses* movies, minus the kidnapping and murder plots. Sister Smelly was only the first of quite a few, who we will get to in due time. You may think that I'm the problem, not them, if I am the one who keeps getting saddled with these allegedly awful people. On some level, yes, it is my fault: sometimes, my chronic health conditions, which are always disclosed fully and up front, can prevent me from doing certain things. I may have to take sick days, I may have to come in late or leave early, I may have an urgent medical test or doctor's appointment, or I may even get hospitalized inconveniently. Sometimes. Most of the time, I excel at whatever I do. I always try my best, even if my best is not the same as someone else's best. If I can't excel, I have the self-awareness to resign. Most of the time, I didn't deserve the cruel treatment that I got. Most of the time, I could have called a lawyer (and have been advised to on various occasions) for the way I've been treated at various jobs because of my medical conditions and personal limitations that have been imposed upon me because of my health. This position was only the first of many where things became problematic, and it only got worse for me from there on out.

Sister Smelly knew that I had rheumatoid arthritis and a suspected case of fibromyalgia. At the time, those and my visual disturbances were my only official diagnoses. She knew about these issues up front, but I'm not sure that she understood the full scope of them — and for that, I don't blame her, because many people do not. Autoimmunity is a difficult thing even for medical professionals to understand or explain, and it is specifically hard for most people to wrap their head around someone who is young having a form of arthritis. It is particularly more difficult to explain when you do not appear to be ill or disabled in any way, when you dress fashionably, have a social life, and are highly educated, intelligent, and ambitious despite your physical shortcomings. But, nonetheless, she knew about my health issues at hand. And I knew, at that time, that something more was wrong. I felt it in my gut, and I feared for the worst. On my lunch break I would make the mistake of Googling my symptoms, and every time I did, Google basically told me I was dying.

One of the teachers' young sons and my brother's roommate had both been diagnosed with cancer that began with shoulder pain. It was shocking and upsetting to me, especially given my cacophony of new symptoms. It ended up being the catalyst that I needed to make a doctor's appointment about all of these new symptoms that included: neuropathy, dizziness, lightheadedness, vomiting, hot flashes, weakness, tinnitus, muscle aches, brain fog, extreme fatigue, and more. I knew that some of it could be related to my rheumatoid arthritis (which, technically was still considered to be "juvenile," though I dropped that term on my own once I reached adulthood and was later formally diagnosed with the "grown-up" version of RA, anyway.) But, I also knew that it seemed like there was more to it.

I made the appointment with an endocrinologist, because I felt that, perhaps, an endocrine issue was at play. Though I wasn't sure that I should have been the day-to-day school nurse, I'm fairly educated about medical stuff, and an endocrine problem seemed like a very likely fit. The day I made the appointment, I found out that my co-worker's son and my brother's roommate were, in fact, one in the same. The two young men for whom I'd been praying turned out to be just one, and his name was Curt. For some reason, that news hit home to me. It broke me down, and I just cried and cried for this boy who I didn't yet know. I went to noon mass on my lunch break that day, and as I sat in the church while old ladies judged me for not kneeling, I felt like the news about Curt was a sign that I was making the right decision in seeing a doctor. It saddened me greatly, but it also scared me to think someone in their 20s could get such a life-altering diagnosis.

I was anxious up until the doctor's appointment. I had to leave work about a half hour early that day, and I'd been reminding Sister Smelly about it all week. Nonetheless, she wasn't in the office to cover for me on time, and gave me a hard time when she did arrive, grumbling and giving me a bit of an attitude. I took it in stride — that was the norm, after all: nice when she wanted to be, seemingly bitter and snappy towards me the other 90% of the time.

I don't remember much about the appointment itself, only that I'd feared the worst. What if it wasn't just a thyroid imbalance? What if I, too, had cancer?

That thought sounds so extremist, I know, and it almost seems like I was making my brother's friend's/coworker's son's situation about me. To be clear, I wasn't — but it did give me a little reality check. Realistically, the idea of cancer isn't far-fetched for people with autoimmune diseases — and it had been tugging at the corners of my mind. Aside from Curt, a friend was also dating someone that summer who had lived through cancer during college. Plus, there was a new warning on my RA medication that said it caused an elevated risk for lymphomas. It was too much of the c-word all around me at the same time, and it admittedly may have caused a mild case of medical anxiety.

However, I'm sure that the majority of people who live with a chronic illness — specifically, autoimmune conditions — have worried about cancer at some point, and maybe even had a scare or two, or at the very least been tested for it via blood work or biopsy. I know I have. Having certain autoimmune conditions puts you at a higher risk for cancer than the general population, as do some of the medications. Many symptoms and behaviors of cancer and autoimmunity overlap, and so do many of the treatments. I've had dysplasias and precancerous cells; I've had biopsies; I've been on a low-dose oral cancer medication and an intravenous chemo drug, both for my rheumatic illnesses. So, the scary c-word wouldn't be entirely out of the realm of possibility for me — and that's what scared me most.

About a week later — on my birthday, actually — I got a call on my cell phone from my doctor's office. I was not supposed to have my mobile phone out when I was on secretary duty, but I'd often place it in the top desk drawer where I could check it if need be.

Of course, I took one trip to the restroom and when I came back, I saw a missed call from the endocrinologist's office. They left a message telling me that some tests came back abnormal and told me to call them back when I could, but left no further info. WHO DOES THAT?

Talk about creating unnecessary anxiety! For some reason, when I saw that missed call, I had a sense that it wasn't going to be an "everything is normal" kind of call. I'd had blood work and a thyroid ultrasound done, and, on top of that, had worried myself sick.

With trepidation, I called back, and because the universe enjoys toying with me a bit, their office was closed for an hour for lunch. Since it was my birthday, I was meeting my mom on my own lunch break for a quick bite. As we were dining, I got a call back from the nurse. The doctor would have to see me in person, but my gliadin-AB antibodies were sky-high, and there was a nodule on my thyroid. The office would send me a copy of the test results in the meantime.

Naturally, this made for a worried rest of our lunch, but I was a pro at investigating the meaning of test results online. When I got back to school, I Googled gliadin quicker than Kim Kardashian would sign up for a selfie convention.

I was more nervous than ever because of the nodule-abnormal labs combo. I glanced at the Virgin Mary statue in the office and thought of my poor coworker and her son, and told myself to man up and keep reading. Luckily, the scary c-word was not what these tests indicated; rather, they indicated a different c-word that would change a lot of things for me: celiac.

"WTF is Celiac?" was my first thought.

I scanned a few sentences of text.

"WTF, I can't eat spaghetti or drink beer?" was my second thought.

This did not make for a happy birthday. Wasn't it ironic that I was being told on my birthday that I couldn't eat cake? As annoyed as I was, though, I felt more relief than anything else. One thing that happens when you live with chronic illness is that you try not to worry people until you have a reason to worry. So, I did not let on to anyone just how nervous I was during this time. I was dropping all signs of leftover Bell's Palsy weight quite rapidly, which was welcomed but unusual, since I was not exercising much or eating particularly healthfully. I didn't tell anyone that I would sometimes go to church on my lunch break to pray and let out a little cry here and there, because I was sick of feeling crappy and having no solid solutions or answers. I didn't tell anyone that I was struggling so much just to get by. So to have an answer that was somewhat manageable was a relief.

The upside to celiac was that it wasn't cancer. This is, obviously, major. The downside to celiac is that, like rheumatoid arthritis and other conditions I have been dealt, there is no cure. There's only a treatment: a lifelong treatment. That treatment is a gluten-free diet. Before that day, I had never in my entire life heard of gluten. Ignorantly, I assumed it had to do with glucose, especially because an endocrinologist who works a lot with diabetes patients was the one who diagnosed me with celiac. That is inaccurate. Gluten is a protein found in wheat, barely, and rye and their byproducts and derivatives. Sometimes, oats and corn are cross-contaminated with gluten. Gluten even hides in places you'd never expect, like prescription drugs, and lipstick, and licorice, and soy sauce.

I took a few minutes to absorb the information I had learned. I waited until I knew Sister Smelly wouldn't catch me, and then called my mom to tell her the news. There wasn't much to share, because I hadn't had a ton of time to do extensive research on it, but I knew that she would be on top of it.

In the months to follow, I would learn a lot about gluten-free living. I found out that another co-worker's son lived with a condition on the autism spectrum and was on a gluten-free, casein-free diet for that. She was a wealth of information and knowledge when it came to eating gluten-free. I was so very grateful for her and all that she shared with me about gluten-free living. I found out that I couldn't "cheat" on this diet. It was for life, and it was very strict. By perusing the National Foundation of Celiac Awareness website at celiaccentral.org, I learned that cheating on the diet could increase my risk for intestinal lymphoma by up to 40%. One study that I found on the NFCA site claimed that a person with celiac - treated or untreated - would be 2-3x more likely than the average person to develop any form of cancer in general. I also found out that cheating on the diet could lead to severe malnutrition and malabsorption, potentially-dangerous pernicious anemia, neurological deficits, infertility, intestinal damage that could be irreversible, and more.

I was eventually diagnosed with acute gastroparesis, gastritis, acid reflux, iron anemia, osteopenia, and pernicious anemia on top of, and caused by, celiac. Most of these things were acute and went away with time; some were chronic and stayed to hang out, still lingering to this very day. Pernicious anemia in particular is a dangerous lack of vitamin B12 in adults. It can cause all kinds of neurological problems and could be partially to blame for my tinnitus, mild upper-register hearing loss, paresthesia, and neuropathy. I was put on weekly B12 injections indefinitely, which I did at home, along with my Enbrel shots.

I was not feeling any better, but I was warned that it would take time. I have gotten five endoscopies and biopsies over the course of seven years, and I still have persisting damage to the villi in my small intestine. Doctors hesitate to call my celiac refractory because I do not exhibit typical refractory symptoms — but it is, at the literal level, a pretty refractory case. Refractory in general terms means that a disease is resistant to treatment. In patients with celiac, refractory cases are often severe and are precursors to cancers and other ailments. So while I thankfully don't have many of the harsher symptoms or realities of typical refractory celiac, my body has not necessarily responded to the gluten-free diet very well, even though I am strict with it. So, my case is technically, on some level, a refractory one. I have tried my best to remain 100% gluten-free, even dabbling in also being corn-free and dairy-free. I also went so far as to formally educate myself on overall nutrition, which has been a massive help in disease management.

As I learned about my new diagnosis, I was still managing and trying to get by. Every doctor's appointment or medical procedure was a thorn in Sister Smelly's side, and the reality of my new life was beginning to weigh heavily on me. I thought of things I'd never thought of before. My decision to enter the field of teaching, which required such commitment and energy (not to mention a strong immune system,) suddenly seemed really stupid. The supplements I took, and candy I snuck, and coffee I drank suddenly seemed like foreign entities who were not to be trusted. Which products could I use? How would I know what to eat? What was safe? Was my shampoo okay? Lipstick? What about Communion at church?

Since I worked at a church, I figured I'd approach Sister Smelly with that particular question. She easily directed me to the right person to ask. We'll call this lady Mrs. Stickupherbutt. Mrs. Stickupherbutt was your typical uptight pearl-clutcher, and looked like she was an aging Stepford Wife just aching to enter her golden years at a retirement home in Boca Raton. Sister was unpleasant a lot of the time. Mrs. Stickupherbutt seemed to be unpleasant 100% of the time. Literally. Remember, I was an English major —so I mean it: she was literally always unpleasant.

"Excuse me," I said, approaching her with a wide, fake smile, and innocent doe eyes, making sure that my top was buttoned up as high as possible and that my cross necklace was visible to her ever-judgmental eye.

"I have a quick question," I said.

"Yes?" she replied.

"Well, I know you are in charge of Eucharistic dealings and the First Communion kids. I recently was told that I have Celiac and I can't have gluten. Gluten is, among other things, in wheat, and I know that the Communion wafers are wheat. I was wondering if you knew about any gluten-free Communion hosts out there? I read about some online," I said.

"Well, no, you cannot use another wafer," she answered. I suppressed an eye roll as she continued.

"To use any other Eucharist is verboten. The Bible says it is wheat," she said.

I questioned the accuracy of her statement, but I'd admittedly never read the Bible cover-to-cover. I thought briefly about my daily devotional and my Bible as Literature class where we covered a good bit of it, but I honestly wasn't sure that the Bible really talked about the Communion wafer at all. Nonetheless, I'd let it slide. I had to admit, her throwing out the word "verboten" in her holier-than-thou tone was a bit intimidating — menacing, almost.

I was angry, though. I was born and raised a Catholic, and while I disagreed with a lot of the politics, along with the church's more old-fashioned and sometimes-hypocritical beliefs and dogma, I had really grown in my personal faith and relationship with God through dealing with illnesses and working at a Catholic school. The Communion was the sacred part of the Catholic mass where I felt the closet to God, and to not be able to receive it was disappointing. Was I going to Hell because I was a Sick Idiot?

"What do you tell parents of young children who are going to make their First Holy Communion but have a wheat allergy or celiac?" I asked. Ha! I got her there. I couldn't wait to see her squirm. She couldn't avoid answering this one.

"I tell them to switch religions," she said aloofly.

I stared at her blankly, in disbelief. How dare she tell me to leave my faith because of a health condition I cannot help!

"What?" I asked, daring her to repeat herself. Her statement honestly left me feeling incredulous.

"I tell the families to switch religions, that they cannot be a member of the Catholic Church, because the child would not be able to receive Communion," she answered. I again speculated that she was probably mistaken or misinformed, but she was in charge of the First Communion program, so apparently this is what she was telling parents of children with celiac disease. It was bewildering. Yet, I couldn't walk away — I just had to know more about this theory.

"Which religion?" I asked.

"Oh, we like to tell them to go Episcopalian. It's close to Catholicism," she answered.

I was amazed at how brusquely she was handling my questions. This was a sensitive topic that dealt with two very personal issues: health and religion. She was suggesting I switch religions the way one would switch brands of toothpaste.

"What if the host was made by nuns and blessed? I thought I read that there were some nuns who made gluten-free hosts," I said.

"They're not. They contain wheat. I know what you're referring to," she answered. (On this issue, she was correct. They were "low-gluten" but not gluten-free. A true celiac cannot eat low-gluten items.)

Deflated, I said,

"Okay. I don't know what I'll do." I had tears in my eyes as I looked at her, waiting for a moment of compassion. I didn't get one.

"Okay," she said. "Back to work."

That's one conversation that I'll never forget having. I should note that in the years since I spoke to Mrs. Stickupherbutt, I have found out that some Catholic churches do, in fact, offer gluten-free Communion, and, if not, that a person who cannot take the host can still go up during Communion and be blessed by the priest. But, nonetheless, that is not all churches, so in some cases, if you are Catholic and have celiac, but still want the proverbial Body of Christ, you're not getting it. You're a heathen that must lower yourself to some OTHER religion. (Insert disdainful sniff here.)

Catholics: you know that whole, "Behold the Lamb of God" part of Mass when we pray, *"I am not worthy to receive you?"* right before Communion? Apparently, if you have celiac, you aren't worthy to receive anything besides banishment to another religion. If you are a Catholic with celiac, the gluten-filled body of Jesus is <u>not</u> your homeboy.

At some point during my illustrious career as school secretary, my bad knee began to get even worse. This was not something that a chiropractor or The Crusoe Fanboy could fix. This unfortunately required another surgery because I could barely walk. It was not really up for debate: I needed surgery ASAP.

Oddly enough, my knee must enjoy acting up around Easter break, because much like the Cathedral incident, my arthroscopic surgery was scheduled to go on around the time that the kiddos would be on their Easter vacation. I would just need to take a slightly longer vacation than the rest of the staff, and would be back at school in no time. I emailed Sister Smelly (who, despite her best efforts to have me type pointless things on an antiquated typewriter, actually had — and could use — email.) I explained to her my situation. During this time period, I was also dealing with the neurological effects of my celiac disease among other things, and was debating being seen at the Mayo Clinic, too, because of the severity of my symptoms.

Her reply was that it wasn't a great time for her. My surgery wasn't convenient, timing-wise. When I gave her a detailed list of the doctor's appointments, she told me that certain days "worked better for her" than others. I didn't know how to respond to these types of comments: I very clearly understood the importance of my position at the school, and could only begin to guess at the complexity of running it. I felt terribly guilty about my absences and the fact that I had to take even more time off for a surgery. But, by that point, I was growing irritated with certain ins and outs of the job. She'd misplace something and accuse me of losing it; she'd ask me to do something, I would do it, and then she would consistently question whether or not I did it; she'd approve something and forget that she had done so; and so on.

In her defense, I think the job was just getting to be too much for her. The main priest was retiring, Sister wasn't a spring chicken, and with the incredibly low budget, she was basically running the school by herself. While I didn't always like her attitude towards me, I did have respect for her in that aspect. What I did not appreciate was her getting snarky with me for "sharing too many details about my illnesses," and then ALSO getting snarky with me when I *didn't* keep her in the loop about something. I could never win. It was always a little too hot-and-cold with her, and I felt to blame for things that were beyond my control. I could not help the shoddy health situation I'd been dealt and I hated when people made me feel like I had to explain it or that I was somehow to blame for it. I always felt as though she didn't trust me, as though she thought that for some unknown reason I would come in late just for giggles, despite having been awake for hours (as evidenced by calls and emails to her in the wee hours of dawn.) It seemed like she thought, for some reason, that I would purposefully schedule QSART tests and MRIs and endoscopies, biopsies, and surgeries during the busy times of the school year with the sole intention of getting under her skin. It was as though she didn't realize the seriousness of my symptoms; it was as though I should have sacrificed my health and well-being for the school — and in retrospect, maybe I should have. I loved those kids and I felt awful about the situation I'd put Sister in. I know that sacrifice is an important part of religion — but this was my body, which is a temple, and I am to care for it. I do know that the Bible at least says that.

But, certainly, she didn't bargain for someone who was frequently coming late or leaving early (regardless of the reason,) and who would get sick in the bathroom while the kids were in class but then plaster on a smile when they were in the office or roaming the halls. I'm sure she didn't expect that her new hire would have to take a medical leave of absence under the Family Medical Leave Act. Clearly, she didn't realize the magnitude of my health situation when she hired me, but, to be fair, neither did I. I'm sure that I was not what she had signed up for. But, guess what? I didn't sign up for the rotten card I'd been dealt, either. The timing may have been inconvenient for her, but it was even more inconvenient for me — who wants to spend their 20s being sick or in pain all of the time? I hated that I was — whether intentionally or not — made to feel guilty for who I was and who God created me to be. But, some religious folks are really good at making others feel that way, aren't they?

Towards the end of my employment at the school — I only lasted one school year — we were barely on speaking terms. The proverbial icing on the cake was when she outright lied to me about the timeline of when she'd decided to replace me and when she (I'm pretty sure illegally) gave unsolicited personal information to a mortgage broker calling to verify employment information with her when she was not within her rights to do so. (I would have made a bigger fuss about it, but we got our house, and so all is well.)

It was a wonderful learning experience and a pretty fun job in general. I loved interactions with the students and their parents, as well as most of my co-workers, but it definitely showed me that, physically, I would be unable to be a teacher. I sadly withdrew from my graduate classes, halfway done with a Master's degree that I was deflated to realize I'll probably never obtain. I have some education credits floating around out there somewhere. I wish I could get a refund on them, but health insurance doesn't pay for lost wages, lost time, or lost dreams, unfortunately. No one reimburses you for the paths that you started on, only to quit because you are a Sick Idiot. If they did, I'd be a millionaire.

The decision was a no-brainer. I wasn't physically cut out to be a teacher, and, truth be told, I'm not sure I have the personality for it, either, unless it was older high school or college kids. (And a later start time.) I'm sure that Sister and most people who know me would agree. Had she shown me just a little more respect, I would not have chosen to out her as Sister Smelly in this book, though I must say that we've exchanged some pleasantries over the years. The school even helped me in a fundraising effort a few years later for which I was very grateful. (And pleasantly surprised.)

Now, please excuse me while I go to Confession to repent for this less-Catholic-and-more-catty chapter.

THAT TIME I HAD SOME (MORE) HORRIBLE BOSSES

It seems only natural to follow Sister Smelly with a few other horrible bosses, who we'll call C-Level: The Stereotype (at Job A,) and Nonprofit Negative Nancy (at Job B.) I am not going to mention their names, the company names, or any specifics, but, these stories need to be told (albeit in no particular order.)

Before I go on, let me say: as you've gathered, I'm not perfect. I'm not a perfect person, I'm not a perfect employee, and, in fact, I don't always do well when I feel overly bossed around or disrespected. For as much as I am not cut out to be a traditional teacher, I am REALLY NOT cut out for corporate life or a regular 9-5-office job. I do better with a flexible schedule and I do better when I feel valued. I thrive as an individual. I don't do well feeling like a number or a sheep needing to be herded. I get bored easily. I don't do well in a rigid environment. I don't do well with workplace politics or office-lady gossip. It's just not me. I don't think that I'm built for it physically or emotionally. So I'm just putting this out there: part of my failures with these companies is my own fault. I can own that. It's hard for me to thrive in that kind of environment, which is amazing for many, but utterly stifling to me. Two of my biggest pet peeves are to feel micromanaged or condescended. I don't appreciate being talked down to, and I also can't stand to feel like someone is breathing down my neck or watching my every move. It makes me uncomfortable. It makes me less productive. It stresses me out to the point of making myself sick. It's just that bad.

However, the way I've been treated at various jobs has been simply laughable and, at times, bordering on cruel. For one, people tend to not take me seriously. I assume part of it is because I don't assert myself. In fact, C-Level: The Stereotype (who we'll simply call C-Level from here on out,) called me into his office one day to tell me that I "wasn't bitchy enough." That says a mouthful. I'm not. I'm just not bitchy, and I will never be able to force myself to be that way. Aside from my being insulted that a man would choose the phrase "bitchy" instead of say, "more assertive," it opened my eyes to one big fact: he didn't respect me.

As for the bitchy: I'm not, and maybe my lack of bitchiness and assertion is why I'm not always taken seriously. Sure, I'm not always great at being on time. And yes, sometimes I get really, really bored during meetings. But, I've always had great ideas and have always been a hard worker with good intentions and a lot of ambition. However, my health problems always seem to overshadow those facts. Being absent at meetings or having to leave work early for a doctor's appointment will always trump the fact that I won a blogging award for the organization, that I got a celebrity to agree to an interview, that a TV show was talking to me about appearing on behalf of the brand, or that, because of me, we got into this publication, or that one. People always choose to focus on the negative. At both Job A with C-Level and Job B with Nonprofit Negative Nancy, my shortcomings (the vast majority of which were out of my control,) very notably seemed to overshadow my achievements. No one, unless they were in my situation, could possibly fathom how utterly disheartening that fact can be. It was a daily struggle to feel not only physically ill, but also undervalued, unappreciated, and often times, practically invisible.

I've written blog posts before about chronic illnesses or disabilities making one feel "less than." Nowhere is this more prominent than in the workplace. For all of the accommodations that these jobs admittedly (though often halfheartedly) tried to make, there was an undercurrent of animosity, distrust, and disrespect that ran rampant. Being sick made me unreliable, or, at least, made me seem that way. My best didn't look like everyone else's best — even when my best, at times, yielded better ideas or better results than theirs did. Different was valued; differently-abled was not. Resentment boiled over amongst coworkers who didn't understand my situation, and many times I would pray that they only understand.

Unfortunately, empathy isn't a skill that is taught in our college business classes, or on the job. If they could only be me for a day, surely, they would understand that I WISHED I could work the same hours as them. I WISHED that I didn't have to come in late because of a doctor's appointment, leave early because of physical therapy, or miss a meeting due to being debilitatingly ill. Both of these jobs allowed for telecommuting, which, naturally, I took advantage of, particularly given my health situation. But there were so many times that I would quite literally cry because I had to spend another day at home. If I wasn't in the office, it was usually because I was ill or had a medical appointment, not because I wanted to lounge around and paint my nails and eat (gluten-free) bon-bons. I usually never call people morons, but anyone who thinks that a life of illness is any way to live is a complete moron. Anyone who thinks that I — or most people — would rather be spending days sick in bed or at the hospital, instead of being productive and working at a fulfilling and gainful job is a moron, or, at the very least, missing a sensitivity chip...big time.

The nature of these illnesses makes it hard for "outsiders" to trust us. My conditions, for the most part, are invisible, so I typically look fine. You would think that this is a good thing, but that's not always the case. Looking healthy confuses bosses and co-workers who are completely ignorant to the severity of the diseases. Looking healthy gives others a pass to inaccurately judge you without taking the time to educate themselves on the seriousness of your condition.

There is also another component of autoimmune conditions that makes it difficult for people to trust you, and that is the unpredictable and ever-changing nature of these diseases and their symptoms. I speak for not only myself but also for the millions of others with these conditions when I say that our physical health can literally change not only from week-to-week or day-to-day, but even hour-to-hour. So you may have seen me laughing and chatting away happily this morning, only to have to leave work early a few hours later due to practical blindness from a migraine, or the inability to type or walk because of a rheumatoid arthritis flare. I could be in the hospital on a Thursday and able to go out to brunch or dinner with girlfriends that Saturday — but God forbid a coworker see me out and about on a Saturday if I called off earlier that week. If that'd happen, I'd be toast. Instead of getting the benefit of the doubt, it would be assumed that I'd be lying. And, on some level, I get it. I understand that it is baffling that someone could be feeling deathly ill one day and perfectly normal the next. I get it that when someone is young and decent-looking and always smiling, that it's hard to wrap your head around the fact that they could be greatly suffering on the inside.

I understand that. What I don't understand is why it has to be that way. I think back to what could have triggered the disdain and distrust I felt from some of my previous bosses. I can never pinpoint it. With C-Level, I had a guess. Once, I had to go to Washington DC to see a specialist. We had car troubles on the way home and the next day my hubby and I had to share a vehicle while his was being worked on. Since I had the option to work from home whenever I wanted to (or so I thought,) I let Mike take the vehicle and decided I would telecommute that day. Typically, I skipped lunch and left work an hour early a couple of afternoons a week to go to physical therapy or to work out, as exercise and physical therapy were crucial parts of my doctor-ordered treatment plan. This day, I decided to go in the morning before I began my (at-home) workday. The gym was within walking distance, and, a little birdie told me that C-Level saw me out walking in the

83

morning and it ticked him off. But there were no lies involved, no shadiness. It was an encounter taken out of context, and instead of addressing me directly so that I could explain, he immediately made negative assumptions, even though I was taking advantage of a work policy that everyone else at the company had equal access to. We were (allegedly) allowed to work from home any time we wanted and also had flex hours and unlimited paid time off, believe it or not, so, it really shouldn't have been an issue. If it was anyone else, I doubt it would have been, but since it was ME, the girl who claimed-she-was-sick-but-really-didn't-look-sick, it gave him a reason not to trust me. And things like that happened often.

There was always an overwhelming sense that he, and others at the company, just didn't believe me or believe in me. I was in talks with a TV producer named Ryan from the now-cancelled *Bethenny* talk show about possibly doing a segment. The show ended up being taken off-air, but there was always a lingering sense that they thought it wasn't ever even a "real" opportunity, that I had somehow fabricated it, or that I wasn't trying hard enough to make it happen. (Truth be told, they wanted me to come on, and not the company's CEO, so, I'm sure that was part of the issue. I mean, why would they send un-bitchy, Sick Idiot Ashley, despite her probably having more experience than him in doing television appearances and public speaking?)

And there were things that went wrong with a vastly under-planned (and under-planned to no fault of mine,) road trip that the CEO was taking on behalf of the company. I worked my butt off trying to get this poorly-planned, haphazardly-executed debacle to come together. I

84

would bring it up constantly and it would always get shelved until the last minute, and yet, there it was: that sense that I wasn't trying, that I wasn't doing well enough, that anything that went awry was somehow my fault, or somehow a lie. They just didn't get it: I was working hard! I wasn't lying! Just because things in my life at times seemed farfetched, doesn't mean that they weren't true. After all, you're reading this book, aren't you? Lots of weird stuff happens to me.

But, boy, did I try to make them "get it!" In fact, perhaps my willingness to over-share or to be transparent was my downfall. I offered to produce medical records or doctor's excuses. I offered to show documentation from the hospital or from the specialist I traveled to see in D.C. I offered to educate the marketing team on my conditions and left the floor open to absolutely any questions they had about what I was living with and how it affected me day in and day out. The problem was, everyone was quick to point fingers and to judge, but no one really cared or tried to understand what I was going through. And I can't say that I blame them: when you live with chronic illness, you learn really early on that you are but a mere speck in this universe, and that not many people care about your problems besides you. That's just life, fair or not.

So, no — no one cared what the reality of my situation was: they only cared that my desk chair was empty, and that I was working from my home office instead of at the cubicle next to them. THAT, for many, was a problem. Sure, I understand the value of "face-time" … but when no one takes you seriously anyway and you're allegedly "not bitchy enough" to fit in, then face-time is much less appealing, to be honest. When you always feel like the enemy, and are made to feel like a nuisance, or like you are less valuable than other members of the team, you're not going to exactly be excited about the days that you do physically go into the office — and I can admit that.

It's particularly difficult when things like this happen:

Coworker 1: "I don't know, we'll have to ask Ashley." (I'm paraphrasing here.)

Coworker 2: "Is Ashley coming in today?" (Paraphrasing.)

Coworker 3: "Probably not, who knows. She's probably sick," she said in a snarky, eye-rolling, venomous tone.

I'm not paraphrasing that one. THAT particular girl? She had zero problem being Bitchy with a capital B — and guess what? She was C-Level's favorite. Go figure. She'll go far in the corporate world because those types always do.

It was actually a case of being not *what* she said, but *how* she said it. The awkwardness after she realized I was sitting right there was stagnant and hung in the air as thick as buttercream. Never once did she apologize for her rude comment; in fact, it was just one of the MANY times she was outright rude to me, yet, never did I get an apology or even an acknowledgement. Granted, I'm sure she was going through her own issues at the time, but that's no reason to take it out on others. I never fully understand why or how grown adults can act that way, but then I simply remind myself that not everyone possesses the same level of emotional intelligence or common courtesy, and that is okay. We all have strengths and weaknesses — I'm just grateful that my weaknesses are of the physical, and not the emotional, variety. I'd rather be a kindhearted and compassionate Sick Idiot than a Bitchy Corporate Barbie. But that's just me.

Little incidents like this occurred frequently. There was one time, shortly after I was handed some new diagnoses, when C-Level called me into his office to feign concern about my conditions and tell me that his friend had lupus, too. He said he knew how hard it could be, but if he knew how hard it could be, perhaps I would have been treated with even the slightest shred of respect. His probing questions about my illnesses seemed invasive and disingenuous. I generally welcomed and even encouraged questions about my conditions, but these questions had a nature about them that was seething with superficiality and ulterior motive, like he was just trying to see if I was going to be a detriment or liability to the company moving forward.

Though I could feel the intent behind his questioning, I answered politely and fought back tears, eventually losing the battle as I openly cried in front of him, much to my dismay and humiliation. But I vowed to not let it stop me. I worked as hard as I could, which was particularly grueling given my health, and while there were attempted accommodations and leniencies that were made during my time at this company, there were issues that showed that the level of understanding and empathy about my situation was extremely shallow. On paper, they had to look good, cover their tracks, and make it seem like I was being treated well. Yet, my workload kept piling on, and I was being dealt further responsibility than what I'd been hired for. That would even be frustrating for a healthy person, but if you see someone drowning, why load their coat pockets with even more stones? This next statement may sound paranoid, but I've spoken to others who have agreed: it was like they wanted me to fail. I think they wanted me to quit — to just give up. That would have been a lot easier for them, with a lot less mess to clean up.

When I first interviewed for the position, I made it very clear that I had ongoing chronic health problems. I put it all out there, so that there were no surprises — I'd learned my lesson from Sister Smelly and I was taking no chances. I told my bosses, the HR guy, and my coworkers. I accepted the job on the basis that I was able to telecommute when I wanted to, that I could work modified hours, and, that I would be able to take advantage of both the company's health insurance and the unlimited paid time off policies. There were no secrets. But that said, to no fault of their own, I believe that they, like Sister, bit off more than they could chew. I do not think that any of us — myself included — realized how much of a challenge it would be. I didn't realize how frequently I'd need or want to work from home or take advantage of flex hours. I could not foresee changes in my symptoms, or the negative impact that such a stressful job would have on said symptoms. I didn't know that, for Christmas that year, Santa would bring me lupus, Sjögren's syndrome, and mixed connective tissue disease diagnoses on top of everything else.

But — health stuff is a slippery slope. They couldn't legally fire me for the limitations that my health problems imposed. They almost had to force me to the point of performance issues so that, if it came to down to it, they'd have a leg to stand on from a legal perspective. I'm not dumb — I knew — or at least suspected — exactly what they were doing. When it was nearing the end, I could tell that a shift was coming. Since all of these people seemed to mistakenly think I was some kind of incompetent ditz, they naturally assumed that I was clueless — but I knew, and it was insulting. The alleged restructuring, the placating tones, the whispers, the alleged policy changes: it was all right in front of my face and very thinly-veiled. The funny thing is, they still didn't have a very good reason to "fire me," as I could counter almost anything they said with saved emails and written proof and documents that I'd saved on my computer and so on. Any areas where I was slipping could be attributed to health issues and I could document that, as well. My positive contributions to the company outweighed the negatives in the eyes of many who worked there — but not in the eyes of those important few. We all know you can't fire someone for being sick, though. So, after the holidays, I was basically "forced to resign." The company outright lied to me and told me that the telecommuting policy changed, and I found out later that it really didn't. They also vetoed a lot of great ideas I'd had while I was there regarding the involvement of affiliations with charitable organizations, and yet, I heard that these ideas become implemented after

I had resigned. So, I guess even though I wasn't quite good enough to keep on board, my ideas still were.

When I was forced to resign, or, rather given the impossible "choice" of having to commit to a regular Monday through Friday, 8am-4pm work schedule, when they darn well knew that I physically couldn't do that, quite a few of my coworkers contacted me about their disgust and disdain with the company and the way I was being treated. I had multiple coworkers suggest that I get a lawyer and many of them claimed that they were saddened to see me go. I didn't encourage any of it, but, the good people who were there saw that I was a good person and a good worker with good intentions, who was simply dealt a bad hand. The whole thing stunk to high heavens and I was asked not to return to finish out my final two weeks because of the "chaos" and discord that my situation was causing amongst my fellow employees.

While it felt good to have people who were behind me, it felt really crappy to have even gotten to that point. I enjoyed the job and the overarching mission of the company. I've seen ideas of mine implemented since I've been gone and it feels both supremely satisfying and flattering, but also like a slap in the face. Instead of finding a way for me to continue working with them, they gave up on me, and it felt awful. Again, it wasn't the fact that my employment came to an end: it happens. People aren't always a good fit at certain jobs or with certain companies. But, the way in which it was handled was just distasteful, and bordering on disrespectful.

I've seen C-Level at various coffee shops or brunch spots since I've left, and I don't even bother to make eye contact with him or say hello. That's very unlike me, but that's just how it is given this situation. I think he knows that the whole thing wasn't entirely fair. I'm not sure if it was him or the CEO who made the final decision, but I felt the same level of distrust and disrespect and just plain fakeness coming from both of them at times. That isn't a good feeling to have, and so, perhaps it's best that this job didn't work out. I don't harbor ill will towards the company or any of my former bosses or coworkers, but there is a touch of bitterness that my potential was clouded by their judgment and my health — neither of which was in my control.

It isn't only the corporate world, though, that has these types of bosses. I worked with a nonprofit organization (Job B) for a while and did a lot of advocacy work for patients with certain kinds of illnesses. When I began, they barely had any social media or blog presence to speak of, and by the time The Incident happened, I had won us some blogging awards, plus many other recognitions and accolades. My role had shifted from community development work to really becoming a peer-to-peer patient advocate and a persona for the organization. My passion was with helping others like myself who had this condition. It was a great job for me, another full-time place of employment that allowed me to telecommute and allowed for a bit more flexible options in terms of working hours. The man who hired me and my former supervisor were both absolutely lovely people, but, once they left, our office went to hell in a knockoff handbag (in my opinion.) The new people who came in were quite obviously pretty clueless about both my own personal health problems and also the health condition/patient population that we served. Their focus was all about fundraising and the bottom line, and their approach was far more businesslike and far less civic-minded and patient-oriented than the mindsets of my previous bosses and myself.

However, although the morale had shifted, I stayed with the job because I so vehemently cared about the cause. I butted heads with the new director (Nonprofit Negative Nancy) frequently. I didn't like her attitude or her personality, quite frankly. When I speak of condescending tones and the fake, political side of working in an office, she is a prime example of what I'm talking about. It was clear that she was there for her rather large paycheck, and not for the cause itself. As someone who, at that point, was only hanging on because the cause, it became increasingly difficult to work together. And while my coworkers there were a little more understanding than they were under C-Level's tutelage at Job A, there was still a bit of animosity and likely some gossip and eye-rolling going on.

One day, I couldn't take it any more. Nonprofit Negative Nancy started lecturing me about how the tone of our blog – the successful blog that I built, mind you – had to change. She knew nothing about blogs, or writing, or social media, and wasn't even well-versed in our cause. I, who am not bitchy, barely argumentative, and rarely stand up for myself, had to argue that I didn't want to change our blog or our social media presence because my whole reason for being there was to help people. I explained that people really needed and relied on the work that we did online through our blog and social networks.

Nonprofit Negative Nancy's reply? I will never forget it:

"It isn't our job to help *those people*," she said.

And yes, she said "those people" like they (we!) were the scum of the earth, like she was some Disney villainess with a curled lip and a snarled tongue. I don't lose my temper often, but I lost it that day. I immediately quit, packed up my belongings, and left. I remember literally shaking with rage. After all, I was "those people" that she was speaking of, and I thought that helping "those people" was, in fact, the job of the entire organization.

I never reported her to the national office and I went on to work with the organization for many years in various other capacities. While I have no negative feelings towards the organization itself, I do not harbor the warmest feelings towards Nonprofit Negative Nancy who, in typical fashion, left and is now the director of yet another unfortunate organization, touting another cause that she presumably cares nothing about.

And as for C-Level, well, I wonder if he thinks that this chapter was "bitchy enough."

THAT TIME IT WAS LITERALLY ALL IN MY HEAD AND I HAD MY BRAIN CUT OPEN

Once upon a time, Dr. McDummy told me that my medical problems were "all in my head." This was simultaneously condescending, annoying, and untrue. If you're a doctor and you're reading this, you should probably realize how dismissive and ignorant such statements sound to patients who are clearly suffering — but also bear in mind that you look even more incompetent when it is proven that yes, it IS all in the patient's head: literally. In the form of a brain herniation.

This is how it went for me. For many years, I'd complain of headaches and other vague symptoms. Dr. McDummy rarely took me seriously and often attributed such symptoms to anxiety or depression. His telling me that my headaches were all in my head (which, let's face it — aren't ALL headaches?) was mildly insulting, but nothing new.

I was suffering, even in the midst of the high highs and low lows of this time period. At age 28, I had recently spoken to Congress on Capitol Hill on behalf of the American College of Rheumatology as a patient advocate lobbying for legislation relating to arthritis causes, which was an incredibly proud accomplishment. But at the same time, I was in pain, and shortly after my wonderful trip to Capitol Hill, I experienced a group of college-aged guys making fun of my limp publicly and out loud in the parking lot of my gym, bringing me down from cloud nine and back to my reality. (It was almost as upsetting as nearly being pushed into the gorilla exhibit at a D.C. zoo during my advocacy trip, but that's a whole other story.)

Primates and arthritis weren't my only problems, though. My migraines had substantially increased, I was constantly lightheaded, and the paresthesia and neuropathy that I was experiencing were getting to be ridiculous. I could barely sleep because of the nonstop ringing in my ears, and I felt weak and fatigued all over. I knew at my innermost core that something neurological was going on. Sure, it could have been the remnants of malnourishment caused by years of undiagnosed celiac disease. It could have even been side effects from one of my rheumatoid arthritis medications. But somehow I just knew that someday something would show up in my brain MRI, one way or another.

I went through the long process that it takes to get an appointment at the Mayo Clinic and, one winter, even flew to their Minnesota hospital to try and find a solution to the puzzle, once and for all. A friend of mine was kind enough to let me use airline points towards a ticket (thanks, Tiffany!) and my mom accompanied me on the trip. After a lot of testing, I returned back to Pittsburgh with little-to-no new knowledge, and my strange symptoms were written off as just another autoimmune issue — a part of the celiac and rheumatoid arthritis disease processes, in particular. However, my headaches began to feel very specific, and very localized to one area. My neck started hurting badly and I felt a really noticeable pressure behind my eyes that was beyond that of a sinus headache or migraine. The increasing intensity of this set of symptoms began to scare me and I decided to investigate even further as months turned to years.

One time, I went to an eye doctor who noticed a "ground-coffee" type pattern in the back of my eye. They recommended that I see a neuro-opthamologist and I grew worried, convincing myself that it was multiple sclerosis or something of that nature. Or, perhaps worse yet, they would find no reason for my new and more intense symptoms, and I'd have to suffer for the rest of my life with no answers and no relief in sight.

I saw the neuro-opthatmologist, who I'd learned was not only one of the best in the state, but rather, one of the best in the country. She gave me a physical exam and pulled up a number of old brain MRIs. The ground coffee pattern ended up being irrelevant and attributed to inflammation, but she did see something else.

"Oh, yes. There you have it," she said, and enlarged the screen for me to take a look. I had no clue what I was staring it.

"I don't know how they missed this," she continued. "You have a Chiari."

"A what?" I asked.

"Arnold Chiari malformation," she said.

I wrote it down and she explained I'd need another MRI to formally confirm it, but she recommended that I see a neurosurgeon. I remember feeling the blood drain from my face. A neuro-SURGEON. Not a plain ol' vanilla neurologist.

I kept my cool, as I always do, but internally, my belly was doing jumping jacks. I was past the point of bringing Mike or one of my parents to most doctors appointments, as I was averaging 1 or 2 appointments per week at minimum, but, that time, I'd wished I wasn't alone.

I don't recall the specifics of the rest of that day, though usually my memory is as sharp as the scalpel that would soon be cutting into my brain. I do remember, at some point, ending up at my parents' house, talking with them and Mike in their living room, and breaking the news that I would need to undergo a combo operation on my neck (laminectomy) and brain (duraplasty.)

It was stranger than fiction. Here I was, newly-engaged and planning a wedding, and now, I needed brain surgery, too. It was November. I was advised to have the surgery sooner, rather than wait until after my June 2011 wedding. It would have likely been far-fetched to happen to me with how relatively small my herniation was, but untreated Chiari malformations can lead to partial paralysis and a dangerous pressure caused by the build-up of cerebrospinal fluid.

So the chaos began. I met with 5 or 6 brain surgeons before finally finding The One. At one point, as my husband and I were driving home after some mundane errand, I randomly made up a rap song on the fly. Apparently when I'm under pressure, I morph into Nicki Minaj.

"My skull's too small, my brain's too big, I need Chiari surgery, I'll have to wear a wig," and *"my brain don't fit, on my spine it sits,"* were some of the finer lyrics.

There was also something in there about *"my head be aching, my vertebrae be breakin', gonna sue some bitches and bring home the bacon"* (because, in the context of this song, I would reap all kinds of glorious financial retribution for doctors having missed the herniation for so many years. I would be able to sue Dr. McDummy for telling me that my symptoms were imaginary. But that was in my fantasy-land where I could rap … it wasn't the case in reality.)

The task of selecting the right surgeon was daunting. I became almost paralyzed with fear over choosing the wrong one. In my mind, there was only one doctor who could be The One, and, basically, I would positively die if anyone else touched my brain. It's not logical, but, brain surgery is a scary thing, and to be thrown to the wolves at such a rapid-fire pace made every decision seem like life-or-death.

I finally settled on a choice who one of my friends (and a fellow *Grey's Anatomy* enthusiast) deemed McDreamy (particularly McDreamy compared to the other candidates.) I focused on enjoying the next couple of months with my family. To me, Thanksgiving, Christmas, and New Year's Eve felt even more sacred than usual that year. Unbeknownst to them, there was still a lingering fear in the back of my mind that something would go horribly wrong during the surgery. I remember having coffee downtown with Mike one day, fighting off the anxiety of the "what-if" scenarios. What if something happened and I was never able to reach my dream of becoming a published author? What if this was my last Christmas? What if I didn't make it to our wedding day? It was scarier than I'd let on.

Mike and my family and friends were great about it, though. I have this Cabbage Patch Kid doll, Winnie, who I have had since my very first birthday. She's been with me to college and at my first apartment and now sits on my headboard at the home I share with my husband and pets in a suburb of Pittsburgh. Winnie's head was beginning to fall off after years of wear and tear, and a lifetime of love. I wrote a popular blog post during this time called "Broken Dolls: The Things and People We Keep, Flaws and All," which explained my upcoming brain surgery and compared my keeping Winnie to my then-fiancé Mike and loved ones "keeping" me despite my flaws and shortcomings. Somehow, Winnie's head falling off seemed to parallel my brain surgery journey, and I became obsessed with fixing her like the doctors, hopefully, would fix me. Even though I was an adult, I wanted her with me at the hospital when I recovered. I needed that piece of home when I awoke after my operation, but I was worried about the fragile state she was in. As brain surgeries go, there was no easy way to fix her, though - like mine, hers wasn't a problem that your average home economics graduate could easily stitch and sew.

I was pleased to discover that places called doll hospitals actually exist for these types of situations. We located one, called Lilliput Doll Hospital, which was luckily only about ten minutes away from our house. I got a quote and, at the time, it was too expensive to have Winnie fixed in time for my surgery. That Christmas Day, though, I received what is still to this day one of the greatest gifts I could have gotten: Mike and all of my family members had chipped in to get Winnie her surgery and presented me with money in a thoughtful card. I promptly cried, as is a typical response from ever-sensitive ol' me.

As it turned out, her surgery would have to be after mine, but the owners of the doll hospital were kind enough to gift me with a guardian angel brooch to take with me to the human hospital, and I still have it in my nightstand to this day.

Unfortunately, on January 2nd, exactly one month before my brain surgery, my brother's best friend Curt, who was diagnosed with Ewing's sarcoma around the same time as my celiac disease diagnosis, passed away due to complications from his cancer. It was devastating for my brother, his girlfriend, and the young man's family and all who knew him. I couldn't think of anything sadder than his situation.

But it was more than sadness that I felt. It was fear laced with anxiety. I naturally knew that it wasn't about me at all, but his death triggered even more emotional turmoil within me than I'd already been experiencing. It was exactly one month before my brain surgery, and all I worried about was meeting the same fate. Of course, it would have seemed selfish to voice these concerns at the time, and so I kept them to myself, no one ever knowing until now how very much his situation frightened and resonated with me. I went to my new church the day of his passing and prayed for his soul, for his family and friends, and that maybe, just maybe, he, along with my late grandfather, Grandpap Boynes, would be able to be my guardian angel in a month as I went through my own lesser, but still admittedly frightening, battle.

The sadness of his passing was inconceivable. I barely knew him and yet felt so tortured by it; I couldn't imagine the deep sadness and loss that his loved ones felt. I felt like I couldn't talk about my fears, though, because doing so would seem tacky and I didn't want anything to overshadow him or his death. Plus, I didn't want to upset anyone any further. At the same time, I also felt like if I spoke about my fears that they'd somehow come to be realized, and I surely didn't want to speak them into fruition. Worse yet, the nagging fear of comparing situations sprang to light. I didn't want to make it seem like I was comparing my situation, though serious, to his, which was obviously far more serious and far more grave. I realize in hindsight that I probably could have expressed these worries and these concerns, and that others would have understood, but I didn't want it to be about me, and I was okay with it not being about me for a little bit.

But it felt awful. It felt awful to know that someone so young, so loved, so vibrant, and who was full of potential and life could just be taken away so suddenly at the cruel hand of one singular diagnosis. It makes you wonder why sickness strikes. Is there a method to the madness? Why do some people become saddled with health problems?

How can our bodies so violently turn against us? How and why can our cells become our enemies? How can the hospitals and the immune systems built to save us also be, in a way, what destroys us? I prayed that God wouldn't force me to leave my family and friends behind the way he asked Curt to do. I selfishly didn't want to be able to relate to Curt's situation any more than I already did. I prayed that my brother and his girlfriend would not have to deal with even more loss if something went wrong during or after my surgery. I sensed that God just wouldn't do that to them, and thank goodness I was right, or I wouldn't be sitting here writing this today.

To be honest, I will never be able to explain why it was that his situation resonated with me in such a way, or why I felt an unspoken kinship with this young man who I barely even knew. In part, I'd always admired his ability to stay positive and strong in the midst of an inconceivable battle. I respected the way in which he enjoyed every moment of his life, and how he truly seemed to live it to the fullest, even while privately dealing with such a serious health problem. I sensed that his friendship blessed my brother and many others who knew him, and I thought, *"that's the kind of person I'd like to be."* He made me want to mope less, and live more. Despite not knowing him, he helped me cultivate an attitude of strength through illness and a sense of positivity through hardship.

My surgery date was nearing. On the weekend before my surgery, Mike, my parents, my brother, his girlfriend Meghan (now my future sister-in-law,) and I all went out for a fun night of dinner, drinks, and games at Dave & Buster's. It was a memory that I'll cherish because it was a lot of fun. There was also an eerie air that enveloped it, though: the unspoken idea that, God forbid, this could be our last outing — or at least our last normal outing — together. If something went wrong during or after my surgery, things may never be the same. I never told anyone, but, to me, it in some way felt like the Last Supper.

On the morning of my surgery, I felt oddly calm. I had selected my own Dr. McDreamy as The One, I had instructed my Mom to hold on to my engagement ring for dear life, and I made sure Winnie was with us. I brought with me my rosary, the guardian angel pin from the doll hospital, and a guardian angel keychain from Ryan and Meghan. I had said a tearful goodbye to my dogs Lucy and Maggie, and I had carefully packed my comfiest Victoria's Secret PINK sweats for the hospital stay. My friends had all called, emailed, or texted by that point, and I had gotten the Anointing of the Sick sacrament at the local Catholic church a couple days before. Members of the United Methodist church I had begun attending prayed for me, as well.

The worst part was saying goodbye to my parents and my beloved Mike. And then the second worst part was the waiting. They hook you up to the IVs and the machines and then you just wait. I'd had knee surgeries and endoscopies before, but this was different. This surgery felt serious and important. I idly wondered about how much hair they'd have to shave, what would happen if they slipped up, and when I'd be able to eat next. I prayed a lot. I thought about food a lot. I wondered if there was any chance that I could lose my memory, or my motor skills, or not wake up from the anesthesia. I wondered how much pain I'd be in afterwards, how much weight I'd gain, if I'd be completely bald, and how big my scar would be. And I prayed. I wondered what would happen if I woke up in the middle of the operation. And I prayed. In fact, I think all I did before the surgery was wonder, and pray.

I awoke, gagging, gasping, and tearing at the breathing tube that was still down my throat. Nurses immediately injected me with some kind of anti-anxiety medication to knock me back out. I awoke again later, this time in the hospital room, surrounded by my Mom, Dad, Mike, and Winnie. I don't remember a lot from that day. I think my Dad took a selfie of Winnie and me, and I assume that there were flowers and Sour Patch Kids at my bedside.

According to my Mom, they had a bit of a scare during my procedure while they waited for my neurosurgeon to come down and tell them everything was okay. They were told that the surgery would last 4 hours. While they waited, they could watch a digital screen that would show them my status from pre-op, to in the operating room, to recovery, each step of the way. A little over an hour passed, and then a nurse came in and called for my family, as the doctor wanted to talk to them. My loved ones said that the 30-second elevator ride was torturous — only to find out that the doctor only wanted to tell them that they finished up a lot earlier than expected and that everything went okay. It was a relief.

The recovery would be a fairly long road, though. I spent a few days in the hospital and had many visitors — some, I remember, some, I really do not. The kind gestures of people coming out of the woodwork in my time of need would not soon be forgotten. There was Courtney, a girl from my high school who worked at the hospital and came by to visit me with balloons and words of comfort, and Laurie, my husband's cousin who also worked there and brought me an elephant Pillow Pet, knowing that elephants are my favorite animal.

My in-laws came, my aunts, uncles, cousins, grandparents, and some of my close friends all showed up, too. Then, there was Ginny. Ginny was a woman who I had only met once at the United Methodist church, Crossroads, that I'd fairly recently begun attending. We had emailed back and forth a few times about my possibly helping with the children's ministry at the church, and she'd found out through word of mouth that I was having the surgery. She came to visit me after only meeting me in person that one time. I will never forget her kind gesture, and it is part of the reason that I eventually decided to join that church. There was a lot more kindness there than there was at the Catholic church where I had the Sister Smelly drama and was told to switch religions because I cannot eat wheat. (Plus, Crossroads serves gluten-free communion! How's that for a sign?) Several pastors from Crossroads also called me during my weeks of recovery, just to check in and let me know they were praying for me. That level of compassion and thoughtfulness will never be forgotten. To me, God was showing me that this was the church where I'd belonged. Even though I'd often eschewed a lot of the politics and dogma that go along with organized religion, this church felt far less judgmental and a whole lot more loving, real, and welcoming than many other churches I'd heard of or been to, and I liked that. I also felt that I just "fit in" there. It gave me great comfort in a time of a lot of uncertainty, and I have continually been blessed by Crossroads and its members to this day, even recently receiving get-well flowers from my prayer group.

Once I was released from the hospital, I stayed at my parents' house where I grew up, and they took great care in helping me to recover. I had friends, old and new, travel from near and far to visit me and bring some joy to my days. Caroline and Nicole sat with me for hours on end; Valerie took me to lunch. My Grandma Boynes was also staying with my parents at that time, and she, along with the both of them, felt like guardian angels on earth. Mike visited me frequently, and I had my pug, Maggie, and pug mix, Lucy, along with my parents' Airedale terrier, Roxie, by my side, too.

My favorite memory from during the early stages of my recovery was when my mom and dad hosted a Super Bowl party. It was actually the day after I was released from the hospital. You'd think that I would have slept the day away, but there was no way I was missing my precious Pittsburgh Steelers in the big game! Almost my whole family was there: my parents, Mike, Nana, Bups, Grandma, my brother, Meghan, and some of my aunts, uncles, and cousins. I remember wearing Steelers pajama pants, a Troy Polamalu jersey, and huddling under a fleece Steelers blanket with my hair in pigtails, letting my long, train-track scar breathe. My face was puffy and my neck was stiff — and I was a little out of it — but I felt blessed to be enjoying that day with some very special people.

It was not always easy, though — I hated the huge scar and the area where they shaved my hair. Plus, I was often in discomfort. On top of the pain, I was easily bored and extremely tired. Much to my dismay, I had to turn down free tickets to a Lady Gaga concert that I was really excited about. But, this period of rest and relaxation gave me time to continue planning my wedding, and to read, write, and recover in a safe and loving environment.

Winnie eventually got her surgery too. She sits on my headboard day after day, a reminder of everything I've overcome since that day when she first came to me, decades ago.

THAT TIME I WENT TO THE OPRAH WINFREY SHOW AND THEN SHE TWEETED ME

In the spring of 2011, I was simultaneously recovering from brain surgery and preparing for a wedding. As you can imagine, it was a stressful time, peppered with occasions of both despair and elation. On a random afternoon in April, one of those elated moments happened out of the blue.

Ever since high school, I had been a fan of the Oprah Winfrey show. I was devastated when she announced that the 2011 season would be her last, and I saw my bucket-list dream of attending her show as an audience member or guest go up in smoke. That is, until that April day when I got a phone call and an email saying that I'd been chosen to sit in the audience at one of Oprah Winfrey's last-ever tapings of the Oprah show.

My jaw hit the floor. Could it be real? I had been on a waiting list for years, and had religiously submitted my information year after year to try to attend the show in some facet. I couldn't believe my luck! I called my mom, excitedly, asking her if she'd join me on the adventure, and, of course, she obliged. You don't say no to Oprah.

I was worried about traveling, but it was long enough after my brain surgery that my doctors gave me the all clear. I remember enthusiastically shopping for an outfit and researching gluten-free restaurants in Chicago. I asked my rheumatologist to give me prednisone to have on hand in case of a flare, and made sure I had all of my post-surgery medications packed, too. There was no way that my health was going to mess up this trip. My mom and I scoured the Internet trying to find out who her guests would be, so that we could try to decipher if we'd get to see a "good" show. We simply had no idea what we were in for, and it was exciting. I would have to be back in Pittsburgh immediately for my May 1st bridal shower, but there was no way I was missing out on this literal once-in-a-lifetime opportunity.

We made the trip to Chicago on April 28th. There was excitement in the air about Kate Middleton and Prince William's upcoming royal wedding the next day, but April 29th had a different meaning to me: it was Oprah day! A part of me wanted to see her interview one of my other favorite celebrities like Justin Timberlake, Britney Spears, Beyoncé and Jay-Z, or Lady Gaga. Or, maybe she'd have a fun tea party to celebrate the royal wedding — I'd be okay with that. I love tea <u>and</u> Kate Middleton! But, really, if we're talking about royalty, I was just excited to see Queen Oprah herself. She inspired me wholly and totally, and I'd hang on every word of every episode as I watched day by day, year after year. To be able to share this fun memory with my mom before I officially got married, especially after all I'd been through earlier in the year, made it seem like even more of a blessing. Plus, there is a part of me that treads on being a little bit "psycho fangirl" when it comes to my favorite celebrities. This kind of thing was totally up my alley. I relish in fame, pop culture, television, movies, music, glamour, fashion, and celebrity encounters. Oprah was like the Holy Grail of all-things-entertainment — and although I was simply a mere mortal lucky enough to be one of her audience minions, I was pumped!

The night before the taping, we dined and shopped in downtown Chicago, and excitedly prepared for the next day. On April 29th, we woke bright and early. We wanted to be among the first in line, as we heard that sometimes seating was first-come, first-served. I had selected a bright floral sundress with a cropped coral sweater and some comfy wedge sandals, complete with a pink statement necklace, as my ensemble for the day. We got ready in our hotel and headed to a small diner for breakfast, excitedly discussing the events that lie ahead.

My mom warned me a few times not to get my hopes up - but I knew that something good was going to happen. Would Oprah invite me on stage to share my story? Would I get to meet one of my favorite stars? Was she going to do one last "Favorite Things" giveaway? What if we won a trip? What if we won a car? The possibilities were endless, and I was only becoming more excited when I began to hear mutters that Lady Gaga had been spotted around town.

After breakfast, we drove to Harpo Studios. We got the obligatory tourist photos outside of the studio, knowing full well that cameras and cell phones would not be allowed inside. That was a bummer, but at least I'd set my

DVR, so that when the episode aired, I could try to spot us in the audience.

As luck would have it, we were only the second mom-and-daughter pair in line, so we would conceivably gain entry into the studio fairly quickly. We made some new friends that morning, chatting away as we waited to get inside. No one knew what our show would be about, or who the special guests were that day. We had heard rumors that the earlier taping that morning was indeed related to the royal wedding, and we speculated that, with it being one of Oprah's final shows ever, ours would be something special, too.

By that point, though, we honestly didn't care who or what the show was about. The excitement of being in that atmosphere was absolutely electrifying, and nothing could ruin the day. Eventually, after hours of anticipation and waiting in line, we were sent into the studio. It is a lot smaller than it looked on TV, but as television studios go, still quite impressive. Being there was breathtaking and exhilarating, and I remember thinking for a moment that I may pass out.

We took our seats and watched enviously as the VIPs took theirs on the stage level. I didn't care though — I was there, and it was beyond amazing, no matter where our seats were. Just as the show was about to start, however, a producer approached us. I was afraid that she was going to tell us she'd made a mistake, that I wasn't supposed to be there. I thought there was a chance that she was the pinch that would awaken me from my dream. But, luckily, I was wrong. She was the bearer of only good news, and hand-selected my mom and me to move our seats even closer.

She led us down to the 2nd and 3rd rows, respectively, and right among the VIPs at stage-level whom I'd been admiring. My mom and I each got an end seat, me in the 2nd row, and my mom right behind me. When Oprah took that stage, just feet from where we sat, I thought I was going to simply combust from happiness. The atmosphere was unlike anything I've ever experienced, and the joy and electricity in that room was tangible. Good vibes engulfed us.

We still didn't know quite yet what the episode would be about, but we'd soon learn. Oprah was doing a scaled-back version of her renowned Favorite Things show, including surprises and giveaways for her audience members. During this taping, we got gifts from Disney and American Express. Jessica Simpson was one guest, and so we got items from her clothing and luggage lines, too. Johnny Depp was another guest, and we got to go with him (yes, *with* Johnny Depp! *And* Oprah!) to a screening off-site at a movie theater. There, we would get a sneak-peek of one of his upcoming *Pirates of the Caribbean* movies. Oh — and guess what? On top of all that, right before we were to depart for the movies, Oprah told us that there was one more guest whose segment would need to be filmed out of order.

It was, in fact, Lady Gaga, and she sang her song, *"Born This Way."* *Born This Way* had become my anthem throughout my brain surgery recovery and all of my health struggles at that time. It reminded me that God doesn't make mistakes, and that I was born this way for a reason. So, as you can imagine, it was hugely moving and inspirational to see and hear her sing it live at that time in my life — especially at the Oprah show. The fact that I'd had to pass up a Lady Gaga concert because of the brain surgery made this occasion seem even more like a "full circle" moment, and it couldn't have been more magical. The "stuff" was good, but seeing Oprah and Lady Gaga (two women who I admire) with my Mom (another woman who I admire) made this an unforgettable experience.

But, my path would cross with Oprah's again, months later. In October of 2011 — on World Arthritis Day, no less — Oprah Winfrey tweeted me. Yes, Oprah Winfrey herself tweeted me personally, on my Arthritis Ashley Twitter account. I had tweeted from the hospital the night before. I can't even recall why I was there, but I remember watching something on the OWN Network from my hospital bed and must have posted a tweet about it. The next morning I awoke to a tweet from Oprah saying to me, "read ur bio. U r a survivor and now in the healing business. Allowing others to 'emerge' from their pain."

Wow. She knew I existed. I was floored that Oprah not only read my Twitter bio, but also felt moved enough to take the time to tweet me about it. For her to call me a survivor and take note of the fact that I wanted to help others to heal and emerge from their pain was one of the most awe-inspiring and validating moments of my life. Maybe, Oprah was right. I was a survivor. Maybe Lady Gaga was right, too: God doesn't make mistakes.

Baby, I was born this way.

THAT TIME I GOT MARRIED AND MY RING GOT STUCK

Most brides want their wedding day to be perfect. It's normal to sweat and fret over every last piece of minutiae. It isn't absurd to pore over even the smallest details when it comes to the big day. Sometimes, though, life throws a wrench in wedding plans. For me, it was the brain surgery and my other health issues.

For the most part, wedding planning went smoothly, except for the unfortunate time that one of my bridesmaids stormed out of the bridal shop (which is comical now — I still love her dearly!) and that other time that I (very maturely) said I wanted to punch my poor brother in the face for innocently teasing me about my hair extensions, which I was admittedly a bit insecure and over-sensitive about. But, though I regret those incidences and some other minor missteps, I wasn't too much of a Bridezilla, and I felt, for the most part, relatively laid back about the whole thing. Stress was present, but it wasn't all-consuming. My entire wedding experience was lovely and beautiful. I relish in those special memories all the time. However, during the process, I would notice here and there that I had to face concerns that, perhaps, the girls in

Bride magazine or on TheKnot.com weren't necessarily worrying about.

It all started when I got engaged in July of 2010. Mike orchestrated the most perfect proposal, on the beach in Treasure Island, Florida, right at sunset. He proposed with the ring in a seashell that, believe it or not, he'd picked off of that very same beach when he was just a child. It was romantic, and we were with friends who captured the beautiful moment in photos. I couldn't have been more surprised. Sheer joy washed over me, followed by perhaps-irrational anxiety because of immediate questions being thrown my way about when the wedding would be, what kind of dress I would wear, and so on. While I was extremely happy and excited, I also became slightly stressed early on, as many brides do. One of my concerns was that I'd really wanted to lose weight, but, if you've ever been on the steroid prednisone, like I had been for my Bell's Palsy and RA, you know that this particular medication makes weight loss a terribly trying feat.

Trying on dresses was most definitely fun, but I felt exposed and insecure in so many of them. I don't know if you can relate to this unless you've been there, but living with chronic physical health problems can really take a toll on the relationship you have with your body. In fact, I'd been diagnosed with secondary body dysmorphic disorder. It was explained to me that my mild case of BDD was in direct relation to my illnesses, and, in fact, that my skewed perception of the way my body looked was because of the way that it often performed: poorly. I hated my body because I felt like it hated me. Years later, I now realize what a miracle the human body was made to be, and I love

115

how strong my body is for always fighting to stay healthy and stay alive, day in and day out – regardless of how it looks on the outside. But as I was trying on those wedding gowns, I didn't feel as physically beautiful or fit as I'd wanted to. I saw prednisone weight. I felt sick and tired on the inside, so I saw sick and tired on the outside. It wasn't feeling like I'd dreamt it would feel to try on those gorgeous gowns. Also, when I found out that I'd need brain surgery, I knew that my dress style and hair styling choices may have to be modified to accommodate the new scar that would be visible as my wedding guests gazed at me from behind. I did not ever share this with too many people, but because of my health, my self-esteem was shot.

I tried to build muscle tone, trim down, and firm up before my wedding, but I couldn't do the same types of exercises that my healthier peers could do, and certainly not with the same level of ease, frequency, or intensity. I grew frustrated at my inability to drop pounds or get into better shape for the wedding, but, more so, I grew upset at my general inability to keep up with others, whether related to fitness or not. I never thought, "why me" or wanted people to pity me, but I did wish that it could be easier just this once, and that my body would just allow me to enjoy the special time that was upon me.

The summer I got engaged, I was also in a dear friend's wedding. I admit, I wasn't the best bridesmaid for her, and I regret that. Because of weight fluctuations that I was experiencing due to medications and periods of activity mixed with inactivity, I didn't want to pay to get my dress altered numerous times, because I just never knew how much puff or water weight prednisone could inexplicably pack on to me. Because of a severe allergy attack on the way to her bridal shower, I was late. And, worst of all, I had to miss her Las Vegas bachelorette party because of symptoms I was experiencing (that I later found out were related to my Chiari brain herniation.)

I felt like I'd let everyone down. She assured me it was all good, but I know that some people involved in her wedding were deeply unhappy with and disappointed in me — perhaps somewhat understandably. But, how could I explain all of that and the fact that I'd also temporarily stopped working a traditional full-time job at the time because of my health, and so my finances were tighter than usual? People don't think about the financial component of a life with chronic illness or disability, but it's a big one. Medical bills and health-related expenses are an unpleasant reality for people with illness, and, sometimes, so is scaling back work hours, either on a temporary or permanent basis. With both my friend's wedding activities and my own going on within that year, money was something to be taken into consideration whether I wanted it to be or not. So was my health.

She ended up having one of the most beautiful weddings that I have been to, and I was so happy and grateful to be a part of it, even learning through her wedding festivities that her sister was a newly-diagnosed fellow rheumatoid arthritis diva. It is somehow simultaneously distressing and comforting to receive this kind of news. On one hand, I'd never wish any illness, especially these kinds, upon anyone — and I wish that no one else ever had to experience the pain and sickness that comes along with them. On the other hand, it is a sad, bittersweet comfort to know that you are not alone. I was glad to know that I wasn't a freak of nature, but I was sorry that she had to go through it at a relatively young age, too.

I told her, like I tell most newly-diagnosed patients — especially the young ones — that most people are never going to be able to understand. The ignorance, rudeness, insensitivity, and mistrust that patients with invisible illness face is otherworldly, and, as a result, sometimes the emotional pain and tarnish that can come with these conditions is almost as bad, if not worse, than the physical.

And the physical was something I was dealing with far too often that year. As I planned my wedding, my hair and my joints were becoming my enemies. We had decided on a beach wedding in Sanibel Island, FL, where 30 or 40 of our closest family and friends would join us oceanside during a sunset ceremony on the beach. Afterward, we'd have a nice dinner and enjoy some drinks. Then, a month later, and exactly one year from the date on which Mike proposed, we would have a somewhat-traditional but somewhat laid-back reception back home in Pittsburgh. As planning went, I was not nearly as stressed as most brides. My health was my main stressor. I think that I knew, on some intuitive level, that wedding stress would likely exacerbate my physical symptoms, and would make the experience more difficult and less enjoyable. After my scary experience with Chiari and the resulting brain surgery, I wanted to live in the now, and to be mindful, grateful, and enjoy each and every day. So, that's what I tried to do. I aimed to savor every little moment as best I could leading up to that very special occasion.

Some moments, though, I'd rather forget. I had a huge scar on the back of my head, plus, my hair had thinned considerably from the rheumatoid arthritis drug that I'd taken for a while called methotrexate. Methotrexate is also used to treat cancer, and, even though my dose was substantially smaller than a cancer patient's would be, I nonetheless had some considerable side effects. Between my hair not growing back over the scar, and my remaining hair becoming thin and brittle, I felt far from pretty, and could only wish that I would look normal and healthy on the day of my wedding. It didn't matter what others saw: I saw sick. I did not see the best version of myself, and that kind of made me sad.

My girlfriends came to my rescue. My best friend Kristen owns a hair salon. She has been a part of my life since we were in Mrs. Checca's kindergarten class at South Fayette Elementary School. Luckily for me, she is also a seasoned stylist, and is one of the few people on earth who I will let touch my hair or do my makeup. One of my other best friends since 5th grade, Caroline, visited me during my surgery recovery and presented me with me money in a get-well card that I was to put towards the cost of hair extensions. Needless to say, these two saved the day! Would I have preferred to have my own, naturally-grown luscious locks styled in cascading curls as I walked the beach in my wedding gown? Of course! But, that said, the glamour puss in me could not complain: hair extensions, though high-maintenance, were fun and looked great.

I also found a stylish gown that had a unique high collar that covered a lot of the scar on the back of my head. Though I still felt self-conscious because of my hair, scar, and perceived prednisone-weight, it was flattering and chic. We called it the Posh Dress. My bridesmaids Kristen and Meghan, my mom, and my maid-of-honor Nicole, were encouraging and positive throughout my experience of shopping for bridal gowns, even when I had mini-meltdowns borne of insecurity. The only problem left, so it seemed, was the unpredictability of my body. I had begun breaking out in strange lesions and nodules from a form of drug-induced lupus caused by one of the biologic infusions I was on for RA at the time. The thought of a wedding photographer taking a traditional ring photo of my hand with these painful red bumps everywhere was upsetting, and it was also one of those small things that the healthy people around me wouldn't ever need to think about. Then, there was the anxiety that came with worrying about a flare leading up to the wedding.

God was smiling favorably on me for my "Victorian tea party" bridal shower and my fun bachelorette party. He allowed my Oprah trip to go without incident, and always seems to send me a good day when I need it most. Though I recall these big events wiping me out for a couple of days afterwards, I was relatively well enough to enjoy each of them and will forever hold the memories close to my heart.

I worried, though, when mere days before we were to fly to Florida, I broke out in a horrible, full-body RA flare. Every part of me that could hurt or be swollen, was hurt and swollen. Between stiffness and swelling, I was the love child of the Tin Man and the Marshmallow Man, and could only rest comfortably on an anti-gravity lounge chair that Mike brought indoors for me to sleep on in our living room that night. I tearfully called my rheumatologist begging for help, which he sent in the way of prednisone and some pain medications just in time for my trip. Thank goodness that the meds worked pretty quickly, and I felt okay to leave for my big wedding adventure.

We got to Florida and things went well. There were very few mishaps, other than a broken nail, an unfortunate bike ride, and lots of no-see-ums (a bug to which I'd never before been accustomed.) It was such a blessing to be with our families and friends all in one place, and to celebrate such a happy occasion together.

The big day came and I couldn't have been more relaxed. I ate a huge breakfast and lounged on the beach until it was time to get ready. At that point, being sick was far from my mind. I was a bride. For once, I wasn't a patient — or at least I didn't feel like one. Of course, my dear friend inflammation, who has taken up permanent residence within my body, had to stop by and wish me a happy wedding day along with everyone else, despite the fact that I'd intentionally left him and his plus-one off of the guest list. During the ceremony, as my husband tried to slip my ring onto my finger, we looked at each other with a cross between laughter and panic. My finger was swollen and it was a bit of a chore to get the ring to fit onto it. I am not sure if anyone else noticed that it was stuck. But, Mike's a strong guy, and with a bit of subtle force, luckily, it slid on (…snugly. And I was not able to take it off for quite some time until the swelling subsided.)

That's just how my life goes — things are never easy, but they always seem to work out in the end. Unlike the ring, when it comes to me, that kind of thing simply fits.

(But I will not be sending Mr. Inflammation an invitation to any future events. You can mark my words. After all, he didn't even bring me anything off my registry, and I'm still eyeing up a KitchenAid mixer.)

THAT TIME I FREQUENTED HOSPITALS AND GOT ESCORTED OFF OF AN AIRPLANE

A lot of people tell me that I simultaneously have the best luck and the worst luck possible. My life sure is a roller coaster in that sense: a lot of good balanced with a lot of bad. Perhaps that balance is the Libra in me. I have gotten used to extremely amazing things happening often times in concert with extremely crappy things. In one day, I could win the lottery and get struck by lightening. That wouldn't surprise me in the least.

So, as luck would have it, 2011 went out on an interesting note. I'd been working on an arthritis-related project with Aleve, and the advertising company they hired had flown me out to Chicago and New Jersey a couple of times. I don't like flying to begin with, but now I have an interesting personal example to serve as part of the reason as to why. First, when I was younger, we inadvertently drove past the site of the US Air Flight 427 plane crash in Pittsburgh. I saw the smoke, while hearing reports of the plane crash on the radio and seeing footage that night on television. That set off my fear of flying — I love to travel, but hate to fly. At any rate, I'd have to get used to it, particularly if I was going to live the kind of life I wanted to live. So, I do it — my airplane trips are often times fueled by mimosas or Xanax — but, I do it. But one night, in December of 2011, I would have a more memorable airport experience than usual. For once, I hadn't indulged in a mimosa and I had chosen to not rely on any anti-anxiety medications. I was exhausted from my trip and, most of all, really just wanted to get home. In fact, I was so tired that I didn't even have the energy to be anxious. The trip had been a nightmare: the crappy, smelly, dull hotel in New Jersey was a far cry from the lush Chicago hotel suite they'd put me up in the last time I'd traveled for this company. I had a small allergic reaction to a hotel soap that contained wheat, and the room smelled like stale cigarettes, which was also an allergy and migraine trigger. So, I didn't sleep well, my meetings were boring, and I didn't like New Jersey. It seemed like a tease to see the gorgeous New York City skyline be so close, and yet be stuck in a crappy part of Jersey instead. I just wanted to go home.

So, as I finally sat on the plane that was about to head back to Pittsburgh, I felt grateful and relaxed. My body had been in extra-sensitive mode over the soap, the cigarettes, and the poor night's sleep, coupled with stress and exhaustion, but little did I realize just how sensitive I was on this particular evening. A gentleman next to me whipped out hand sanitizer as we backed away from the gate and proceeded to get into line for takeoff. Almost immediately, I felt a rash begin to form on my face and my chest. I thought that my lips and throat felt itchy, but I was sure it had to have been my imagination. You couldn't have an allergic reaction to hand sanitizer just by breathing it in, right? I tried to reassure myself and made the mistake of gripping the armrest that he'd just touched with his freshly-sanitized hands. My arm and hand grew itchy, splotchy, and red almost immediately. I began to feel like I had trouble breathing and broke out in welts and hives. A flight attendant rushed towards me and promptly called over a colleague. Together, they looked at my rash, hives, red nose, watery eyes, and swelling lips, and agreed that I had to get off the airplane. So, much to the dismay of all the passengers on the full flight, the pilot made an announcement that we had to turn around and go back to the gate. Being that we were next in line to take off, the dirty looks I got as I stood could have melted Elsa's *Frozen* kingdom. I was absolutely humiliated, particularly when the flight attendants escorted me off the plane and plopped me down on a wheelchair, as paramedics hurriedly pushed me through the airport to a little makeshift infirmary area. Luckily, with an IV and some steroids, Benadryl, and oxygen, my allergic reaction was under control. They put me on the next flight home to Pittsburgh and I slept the whole way home.

However, after that incident, the rest of 2011 went swimmingly. Heading into 2012, I was feeling positive. I had recently been named one of Pittsburgh's Top 40 Under 40 and attended an amazing gala where I was honored along with the other recipients. I made appearances on TV and in magazines, and received a lot of great opportunities that came out of the designation. My husband and I took an amazing trip to New York City — by far one of my favorite places on earth — right after

Christmas and we were ready for 2012 to be my year. I'd recently finished writing my first fiction novel, called To Exist, and between that and 40 Under 40, it felt like good things were up ahead for me.

After we arrived home from NYC, I was scheduled for an intravenous infusion of a new biologic drug. While biologic drugs often work wonders for most people, I have a chemical sensitivity that causes me to be extra-sensitive to pharmaceutical drugs and certain manmade substances. I am one of those people who almost always gets side effects from and reactions to just about everything, even the mildest of medications. So, I'm not bashing these drugs, by any means — they work well for so many patients, and are a saving grace for a lot of folks who suffer with autoimmune conditions. But, this is my memoir, and my story alone, and my personal story happens to involve problems with a lot of drugs, unfortunately. Remicade had caused me to have drug-induced lupus, and Humira made me have uncontrollable spasms in my arm, as well as shortness of breath. I'd long gone off Enbrel due to a black box warning from the FDA coinciding with an infected injection site and increased headaches, which were nonetheless later attributed to the Chiari. I felt hopeful about the new one I was trying, called Orenica. It was an infusion like Remicade and it felt like a fresh start, especially given its proximity to the new year.

As always, I dressed in comfortable sweats (this time, rocking my new pink and purple Under Armour hoodie that I had just gotten for Christmas and was obsessed with,) and loaded up my Michael Kors tote with my iPad, some fashion magazines, and a book. I had gotten infusions before, so there was no foreseeable reason for me to bring anyone along with me. I knew what to expect. Though I'd be a little drowsy from the Benadryl they'd give me as a pre-medication, I was sure that I'd be able to make the less-than-10-minute drive from the infusion center at the hospital back to my home. It wasn't a strong enough dose to make me feel necessarily all that loopy in any way.

I checked in and chose the recliner that looked comfiest. In the old infusion center, I would take the one that was near a window, away from the registration desk, and close enough to see and hear the TV without being practically on top of it. This was my first visit to the fancy, upgraded infusion and oncology center, and so my recliner had its own personal television, was heated, vibrated like a massage chair, and had a beautiful lighted mural on the ceiling above me. If I didn't know what I was there for, I'd say that it was like a spa — or at least it felt like one in comparison to the previous and notably more dismal infusion center. As usual, I asked the nurse for extra blankets and a ginger ale, because I often got nauseous with my infusions.

He brought me both after what seemed like an eternity of waiting. I have nothing against male nurses, of course, but was disappointed that he was the one who would be helping me that day. I'd never had him before, and I'd built up a sort of camaraderie with the other two female nurses who had attended to me in the past. But, he was a nice enough guy who lived near me and liked to talk about his cats. I'm just one of those people: if you bring up your animals, and get me talking about mine, we're instant friends.

The infusion went a lot quicker than I'd anticipated, but was without incident. I live just 4 miles away from the hospital, and I was looking forward to getting home, posting a blog for work, and then snuggling under my blankets with my pug, Maggie, and my cat, Jack, watching chick flicks for the rest of the day. However, on my drive home, I felt extremely lightheaded and dizzy, and slightly short of breath. My hands felt numb, and I worried that maybe I shouldn't have been driving. I pulled over, and reasoned with myself. It had to be anxiety or just a little woozy feeling from the meds. I'd be fine.

After a moment on the side of the road, I decided to give it another whirl and drove home. When I got home, I let my dog out, fixed myself a cup of hot tea, and went straight up to my office where I promptly lit a scented soy candle and sat down at the computer. At this time, I was working from home and was on a deadline. I had to get a blog posted by the end of the day, regardless of how I'd felt.

I began to type away, and — I don't know how else to explain this — it felt like my heart stopped for a second. I panicked as I stood up and felt my brain and my stomach drop to my knees. I took my pulse hurriedly. My heart rate had to have been above 150. I tried to settle myself by taking deep breaths. I saved my file, blew out my candle, and my dog and I headed downstairs. I could tell she was worried as she stared up at me with her beautiful, bulging pug eyes. I debated my options. I could wait a couple of hours until my husband got home. I could call my mom or dad, who were working, but would probably be able to come over if I needed one of them to do so. I didn't want to bother anyone, and I didn't really know my neighbors enough to have one of them come over and sit with me. I tried to tell myself it was just anxiety, but, somewhere, in the pit of my stomach, I knew that it wasn't.

I felt another "drop" sensation. I immediately grew flushed and my heart felt like it was going to beat out of my chest if I didn't pass out first. I simultaneously had to vomit and pee. My stomach began cramping intensely and I had sharp pains in my neck and chest. I decided to do what I'd never done before: I dialed 911. This was not how I had envisioned 2012 starting out.

Two policemen arrived at my door. They sat with me until the ambulance came. I tried to remain calm and comfort my pug, Maggie, who, at this point, was very agitated and upset. My little best bud Maggie is a sweet dog — towards me. Ever my sidekick, I love her dearly, and am so grateful to a former work colleague named Allison, whose family I adopted her from. When we got her she was named Mitzi, but Mike and I decided it didn't fit her. We renamed her Maggie, but we jokingly still refer to her more naughty alter-ego as Mitzi.

Mitzi was surely out in full force that afternoon in my living room. While Maggie a.k.a. Mitzi is sweet and loving to me, she is not necessarily kind to strangers, particularly if they are men and/or enter our home through the front door. Focusing on her not attacking the police officers was a nice distraction from the intense physical discomfort and sense of fear that I was feeling at the time. Plus, I took solace in the fact that she was such a strong protector. I also have a sweet, loving, big, dopey 95-lb Doberman named Brutus (who wasn't yet around during this adventure) who looks tough and scary, but truth be told, Maggie/Mitzi is the true guard dog. She's possessive of me, super-protective, and neither these policemen nor this illness was going to hurt me that day. She would make sure of it.

I was the picture of calm on the outside, but on the inside I felt like something was terribly wrong. The paramedics came barging into my house and took my vitals. They agreed that something was awry and told me we'd have to go to the hospital. They loaded me into the ambulance and hooked me up to a heart monitor. My heart rate was nearing 200. Everything started to become a blur to me. I heard them radio in to the hospital and mentioned the words "possible heart attack" either to the dispatcher or amongst themselves. That didn't help matters much, and I watched in frustration and fear as my brand-new Under Armour hoodie was literally cut right open with scissors.

"We're going to have to give you a shot that is going to stop and reset your heart. It's going to feel very scary, but we need to do this to get it into a normal rhythm, okay?" one of the paramedics said to me.

I do not recall my exact reply, but I do recall that I demanded for them to get ahold of my husband and/or parents. I also recall being really, really bummed about my new hoodie being cut open.

He wasn't lying when he said that the shot would be scary. Unless you've been injected with adenosine or something similar, I really can't describe the sensation to you. When they say that it stops your heart for a second, they aren't lying. I truthfully cannot think of anything I've gone through in my life that's been more terrifying than the few times I've had adenosine administered to me.

It did the job, though my heart rate was still higher than it should have been. When I got to the hospital, they hooked me up for more tests. They ruled out a heart attack, and had no explanation for my symptoms. Eventually, they deemed me okay to go home, despite the fact that I was still having tachycardia, feeling lightheaded and flushed, and experiencing both bowel and urinary urgency.

Unfortunately, this wasn't a "one-and-done" situation. The second time I had to call 911 was on the way home from Sunday dinner at my parents' house. I had Maggie with me, and Mike was driving in a separate car, a few minutes behind me. I had to pull over because a similar episode occurred. I called 911 and the ambulance came, but I wouldn't let the paramedics take me away, out of concern for my dog. Later that night, after I made it home safe and sound, my husband had to drive me to the emergency room for the first of countless visits. This time, they ended up admitting me for observation. I underwent test after test. After a few days, they finally ruled out a serious cardiovascular problem, but still couldn't pinpoint exactly what was wrong. Most doctors agreed that this wasn't anxiety. There was something physical going on that was causing a heap of symptoms, and any anxiety that

I had was in reaction to the physical discomfort I was in and a rational fear of the unknown. Eventually, after about 4 days, they sent me home. I'd have to fill jugs with urine so that they could rule out a carcinoid tumor or pheochromocytoma. In fact, while I was in the hospital, a doctor prepared me that one of these two conditions could be a real possibility, and even gave me a pamphlet about "dealing with serious disease," since it was rather likely that I would have to do so, and, to some extent, had already done so for years.

But — yeah, that was real comforting. Give the Sick Idiot a serious disease pamphlet, then send her home. Makes sense.

They also sent me home on a heart monitor, even though they were "pretty sure" there was nothing wrong with my heart. Another great comfort: to be told they're "pretty sure" when it comes to arguably the most important organ in your body.

The next month or so was a nightmare. I had made a few more ER trips, gotten a few more shots of adenosine, and had a few more doctors scratching their heads. After a particularly bad spell the night of the Super Bowl that year (another ambulance ride, this time, in a snowstorm,) I was admitted again. I underwent several of the same tests, eventually ruling out a carcinoid tumor, pheochromocytoma, a heart attack, and mastocytosis.

The days all began to feel the same. Almost every day, my dad would visit me during the day, and I appreciated it more than he could ever know. Sometimes, my friends Val and Nicole would stop by. At night, Mike and my mom would come, and on a few occasions, my other family members would pop on in. I received cards and flowers and gifts from friends, family, church members, and even some strangers who followed my journey online. In the midst of all the chaos, there was that simple truth to hold on to: people were innately good. It was nice to know how many people truly cared. That is one glimmer of hope and goodness that sparkles brightly when you deal with health problems: when times get tough, there are always people around you — even people who you may not think of or even know of — who are rooting for you, praying for you, and who are inspired by your story. You never know who is going to show up for you, who will be there in your dark moments, or whose life you will touch simply by sharing your journey and living your truth.

Eventually, I was released from the hospital for the second time throughout this experience, but would be hospitalized once again before it was all over.

Oh. I forgot to mention…

While this was all going on, I had also been nominated for the Leukemia & Lymphoma Society's Woman of the Year campaign — and, because I'm apparently a crazy person, I accepted. Total Sick Idiot move. Why I thought that was a good idea given the timing was beyond me. So, there's me: hospitalized three times for four or five days a pop, while also embarking upon a campaign where I am expected to raise thousands of dollars. That seems logical.

So in the midst of 911-calls, hospital food, ambulance rides, hoodie-cutting, and filling up jars with my pee while rocking a heart monitor, I was also planning several fundraising events, composing a letter-writing campaign, and cold calling potential donors. I planned a "dog party" fundraiser, a wine-tasting fundraiser, and a girls' night out spa party for charity. I enlisted the help of friends who donated proceeds from book sales or salon tips or happy hours to my cause. I sent hundreds of letters, and even more emails.

I may have had to go to the ER immediately following the dog party. I may have been wildly sick the night of the wine tasting. I may have had to cancel a TV appearance and a speaking engagement at our local service summit. And for one happy hour, I may have only lasted about 30 minutes before having to head home. But — I did it. In just 10 weeks, all while being quite sick, I raised $11,000 for children with pediatric cancers, in memory of Curt. I've got to say — that felt good. It felt good to be able to achieve something positive, even in the midst of illness.

As fate would have it, my fundraising efforts raised my online profile even more, and, a follower of my Arthritis Ashley page took note of both my efforts and my struggles. Her daughter, as it turned out, had been having a lot of mystery symptoms similar to mine. She saw a translational medicine specialist in Washington, D.C. — a rheumatologist who took a more integrative and whole-body approach to managing these types of conditions. He was pricey, and it was difficult to get an appointment, but it would be worth a try.

Despite all of my ER trips and hospital stays, I'd come up with very few answers. The lack of results and solutions was both baffling and ironic, considering that Pittsburgh is home to some of the best hospitals in the country, and, according to some, the world. One thing that came out of all of this was that I was formally diagnosed with POTS and hypotension. Hypotension is low blood pressure. POTS is postural orthostatic tachycardia syndrome, and is an issue with the autonomic nervous system. Some of my ER trips had elicited mention of the potential involvement of my autonomic or sympathetic nervous systems, and so, this made sense. But, nonetheless, I wanted to know the "how" and "why" behind the diagnosis. What causes this condition, where a person's blood pressure drops and heart rate goes up simply from standing or changing positions? And how can it wreak so much havoc?

After careful consideration, and a lengthy process to be accepted as a patient there, my husband and I decided to travel to D.C. to see this mysterious doctor. For privacy reasons, I won't give out his name, but we affectionately nicknamed him Bobo, and I refer people to him all the time. This guy was a true godsend. He has worked with the National Institutes of Health and the Arthritis Foundation. He has done a lot of research and is quoted in many medical journals. To be in his presence felt like an honor.

We went over my extensive health history and I brought with me my various inches-thick medical files from various doctors. I got 32 various-sized vials of blood taken that day (which had beat my old record of 18 at the Mayo Clinic. If vampires were real, I'd be a living, breathing Starbucks to them. Step right up for your venti vampire latte, made with real Sick Idiot blood! Substitute plasma for a small upcharge!)

After a few weeks, my results were in. We did a phone consult and I learned a lot. He was so patient, kind, and respectful. I enjoyed talking with this doctor because he was never preachy, patronizing, or condescending towards me, and often spoke to me almost as though I were a peer.

I learned a lot in that phone call. For one, my blood is apparently a bit more viscous, sticky, and clot-prone than the average healthier person's. He said that he has found this kind of thickened state to be common in patients like myself. Even my red blood cells were a bit cystic, and these cysts were potentially formed by protozoa and biofilms in my system — again, common in folks with autoimmune or inflammatory diseases according to him. My thyroid levels were in the normal range but one component - my T3 - was slightly off. My inflammation markers and markers for celiac disease were unsurprisingly sky-high, and of course my ANA and rheumatoid factor were off-the-charts positive. On a good note, it didn't look like I had any immediately urgent or life-threatening problems. On a bad note, fixing me would be a time-consuming journey to say the least.

Dr. Bobo recommended quite the laundry list of natural supplements coupled with prescribing traditional pharmaceutical drugs. I loved his integrative approach of Western medicine mixed with a holistic regimen. One of the supplements, Bolouke Lumbrokinase, has inexplicably been a lifesaver to me. It's rather pricey, and so, there's been times I've been tempted to skimp on it, or skip it altogether, but I've noticed that whenever I do go off of it, that I end up back in the hospital, so … lesson learned.

To this day, I continue with some of the treatments that Bobo recommended. I guess that, contrary to popular belief, some problems can get solved in Washington, D.C, after all. (*even if I did end up in a random Frederick, MD hospital on the way home.)

THAT TIME I WENT INTO REMISSION FOR A LITTLE BIT

Somewhere along the line in 2012, I went into remission — and stayed there for a good while into 2014. Often times, children who are diagnosed with certain forms of juvenile arthritis go into remission by the time they are 18, or, at the very least, before they turn 21. Sometimes, it's clinical remission where the disease is dormant and they even can go off medications. Sometimes, it's drug-induced remission, in which case, the pharmaceuticals are causing them to be symptom-free, and they'll stay on the meds in order to stay in "remission." Either way, some of these folks will go on to live healthy lives and won't ever be bothered with the likes of juvenile arthritis again. Many others will remiss for a few years, and eventually develop adult-onset rheumatoid arthritis or a related illness down the road. I never went into remission, at least, not until I was 29 years old.

I really couldn't believe it. Granted, I still had my celiac and chronic migraines to contend with, as well as some neck and knee pain lingering from my surgeries, but my RA symptoms and other hallmarks of any kind of rheumatism were all but gone. My labs had normalized. My inflammation rate, and white blood cell count, and even RA markers were completely, utterly, unremarkable. I had blood test after blood test come back as "normal" or "negative" — something that I had not really ever had experience with up until that point.

It felt like I was living a dream: I was taking kettlebell classes at the gym where my husband teaches, we were going on 20-mile bike rides, I was going to Zumba classes regularly, and I had even started to like the way my body looked and felt. I joined an online fitness program and took yoga classes all the time. Fitness became part of my identity whereas before it had never been much more than a fantasy or an afterthought.

I eventually decided, at the urging of a very talented author and health coach, Ms. Lindsey Smith, to enroll at the Institute for Integrative Nutrition to become a certified holistic health coach. I had been helping and educating my fellow patients for years already as Arthritis Ashley and through my peer-to-peer outreach and patient advocacy work. I was already fairly knowledgeable about nutrition because of my celiac disease and a general personal interest — why not take it a step further?

After the great success I'd had with Dr. Bobo and a mostly-natural approach, it seemed that integrative medicine and learning about nutrition could be a good fit for me. I enrolled and spent the next year immersed in coursework about nutrition, life balance, natural wellness, and different dietary approaches and theories. I learned about the bio-individuality of the body and it began to make sense why the traditional pharmaceutical approach did not always work for me, but did work well for others. It was because we are all biologically different and we all have unique backgrounds and genetic makeups. I began to learn that how we think is almost as important as what we put into our body. And then, suddenly, I knew what I had to do: go *au naturel*. (Just not in the whole "naked" sense of the phrase.)

Eventually, I went off all prescription medications. Sure, I was on a crap ton of supplements, but, my approach was all-natural. I stayed gluten-free, and also toyed around with other approaches: paleo, Mediterranean, pescatarian, vegetarian, and so on. It just made sense. I incorporated acupuncture, massage, reiki, yoga, and chiropractic into my treatment plan. I did a lot of fun things while I was in remission: went horseback riding, rode bicycles on the beach, went white-water rafting, did a zip lining and ropes course, and worked out almost every day. I even participated in a kettlebell competition.

I learned that I had potential intolerances and allergies to a plethora of various foods, and I read a lot of books about health coaching and nutrition.

One time, I decided to "test" if being gluten-free was even necessary. Perhaps they'd misdiagnosed my celiac disease! I don't know why I thought that could be the case, or why anyone thought that this was a good idea, considering that I'd cried (real tears) more than once about being accidentally glutened at restaurants and parties. But, I was feeling so healthy and almost invincible that I figured it would be worth a try.

"Why not test my body's limits?" thought the part of me that lacks common sense.

For some reason, my doctor said to go ahead and give it a try if I wanted to, even though we all know that people with celiac aren't supposed to cheat. Ever.

So, "give it a try," I did. I decided that I'd do it on a Friday, and I created my menu of "naughty" foods. Oh — I didn't just choose foods with gluten — I chose the worst of the worst. I mean, health coach or not, if I was going to get a free pass to indulge in all of my guilty pleasures that I hadn't eaten for years, I was going to take advantage of it. On Friday, I would have cheese tortellini, wedding soup, and bread sticks. I would also have some Twizzlers and the French shortbread cookies from Starbucks. If I was still alive come Saturday morning, I would have some sausage gravy over biscuits from a local diner for breakfast, and Pizza Hut thin crust pepperoni pizza and a Corona for dinner. (This was back when I still ate meat.)

A few months earlier I had accidentally eaten pasta salad at a party, thinking it was gluten-free potato salad. I then threw up for hours on end. This should have been a good indicator that this adventure into gluten gluttony would not end well. And it didn't. I did not make it past my Italian dinner, which I regret, because I still regularly and intensely crave Twizzlers, and gravy with biscuits. But, that night, all of my really expensive supplements ended up bidding me adieu in a steam of vomit.

Again, I say: lessons learned. We can't win 'em, all, but I did learn that my celiac DEFINITELY didn't go into remission along with the rest of it — and even if it had, a true celiac can never eat gluten. Ever. I made another mental note of this fact.

At any rate, my remission didn't last, anyway. My RA isn't as bad as it used to be, but it got bad enough again that I decided to try the chemotherapy drug, Rituxan. The anxiety I felt about going back to that hospital for infusions was daunting. While nothing bad happened as a direct result of these chemo infusions, it did not help my symptoms, and I have had widespread, deep set flu-like bone aches ever since. That was 6 months prior to me writing this. I'm now back on weekly Enbrel injections, along with Botox for Migraine every 3 months, but most other stuff that I take on a regular basis is still natural.

Each day, I do my Bolouke, plus a supplement for migraines, a supplement for hair growth, my JuicePlus+ capsules, prescription Vitamin D, Vitamin B12 sublingual tablets, Vitamin B12 weekly injections, liquid B-Complex sublingual drops, a garlic tablet, turmeric compound powder, chromium piccolinate, Osteo BiFlex for Joint and Muscle, and more, including various homeopathic sprays and tonics. I also drink a nutritional meal-replacement shake each day, regularly juice fresh fruits and veggies, use a special migraine headband, and do earthing (a.k.a. grounding) treatments. I use essential oils, both topically and as aromatherapy. I get a deep-tissue massage once per month, and acupuncture as needed. On a particularly bad day, I'll rely on the steroid prednisone and/or a muscle relaxer and/or a narcotic pain medication Sometimes I need additional drugs or trips to the hospital for bad migraines. I'll take over-the-counter medications to try to control allergies or reflux as needed. I sleep with a humidifier, a special air filter, and allergen-free bedding. My heating pads and Epsom salt baths are my best friends at night. Sometimes, I need a dose of Zofran for nausea here and there — and this entire regimen could change by the time this book goes to publication. It is not a perfect solution — I wish I was 100% natural and/or completely cured — but I'm trying to get to a place of balance, and a place of healing, and hopefully reach my status of "remission" once more. What I've learned, though, is that what works for me may not work for the next person. I've learned that we must practice self-care, that we must educate and advocate for ourselves, and that we must always listen to our bodies. It is also important that, as patients, we talk to our doctors before starting any new medical treatment, drug, or exercise program.

I can only speak from my own personal experience, and view life from the sometimes-paradoxical lens of being both a patient and a health coach. I'm not a doctor, so I can't give medical advice, but I feel that I can at least advise you all to be your own best advocate and to take care of your body: it's the only place you'll ever have to live.

As of 2012, I am a certified integrative nutrition health coach, and a board-certified drugless practitioner, and am in the process of also becoming a certified international health coach. After all, I like to help others (particularly those with similar health struggles) to take charge of their wellness, learn to love their body, and try to find peace with their journey … even if, like mine, it isn't perfect.

THOSE TIMES MY ILLNESSES CAUSED INTANGIBLE TURMOIL AND I ENCOUNTERED SOME INTERNET TROLLS

There are a lot of incidents — little and big — that my life with chronic illness has either directly or indirectly caused, or, at the very least, affected. From friendships and relationships to everyday interactions with strangers, there are a lot of nuances about life with chronic illness that are difficult to navigate or explain.

If you live with an invisible illness, people tend to judge you. I've had to use a handicapped parking pass all of three, maybe four, times in my entire life — and for good reason. The rude stares and perceived judgment I received while doing so has made me never want to use it again — and I haven't. I would never use it unless I absolutely had to, but it's sad that the reactions of other people is a part of why I would ever hesitate, even if I needed it. I get it that I'm not in a wheelchair, but the public needs to understand that disabilities can come in all shapes and sizes, and that illnesses can be mind-blowingly invisible. It's also upsetting when you get stares as you're limping through the mall, or when people comment on your lupus butterfly rash without provocation.

Much like the ignorance of these folks and of various coworkers and bosses, there's also a surprising amount of ignorance from medical professionals. You'd think that, being in the healthcare profession, they'd know a little more about these conditions, or at least wouldn't suffer themselves from Foot-in-Mouth Disease. Aside from all of Dr. McDummy's screw-ups, I've had doctors, nurses, and medical assistants say things like:

"Are you sure you have RA?"

"You're too young to be getting a bone scan."

"Arthritis? At your age?"

"White people don't get lupus."

"Is gluten sugar?"

"People with RA don't usually take chemo like this."

"You certainly didn't have your C1 removed or resected, either in part or in entirety." (He changed his tune when I showed him the x-ray. Yes, I did, sir. I was there. My C1 is not.)

I've had pharmacies give me medications containing gluten and tell me that it won't harm me; I've had chiropractors try to sell me wheat-containing supplements that the manufacturer said are not gluten-free or safe for people with celiac disease. (And boy, did he continue to rudely argue with me about it, nonetheless!)

Then, there were the times that were more hurtful on a personal level. I've had friendships destroyed because of my health — again, either directly, or indirectly. In college, for example: I admittedly wasn't a great roommate. I'm just not a roommate person to begin with, but I was also very sick at the time, and often isolated myself because of it. I was living underneath a huge, debilitating brain fog because of my Chiari, and I was continually being fed medications (for example, antidepressants) that were making things worse because they weren't needed and the true issues (like Chiari and celiac) were undiagnosed. I forgot to do things around the house or call people back, I was late to things, I missed certain events or special occasions, and unintentionally made poor choices. I eventually became antisocial because I felt ostracized from my peers and largely misunderstood by my friends. It seemed that no one ever saw my reality or my intentions, and I did nothing to paint my situation in a more positive light. Like most college kids, I went out, I partied, I tried to have fun, but I was not fully aware of my health problems or even who I was as a person. As with most people that age, I also had some maturing to do. I think it was easier for people to write me off than to truly try to empathize or understand. I felt homesick on top of being physically sick, and the endless frustration of undiagnosed yet serious health issues at such a young age was weighing heavily on me, affecting my grades and my friendships.

I became very introverted and, by proxy, a little bit selfish. I was largely tuned-out to things that my friends were going through because my own problems seemed to be massive and consuming. To shed some light on it, when a person has undiagnosed celiac disease, it is as though their body is literally starving despite getting enough to eat. I was constantly malnourished, and, as a result, tired and "foggy." Though I don't usually harp on the fact, it can become very serious, and, for some people, even life-threatening. Unnecessary medications due to misdiagnoses, coupled with normal college-age antics and drama led to a not-so-healthy dynamic between my peers and me. I felt very left out, and they, in turn, probably felt like I was purposefully distancing myself from the group or somehow being shady or dishonest. Plus, I was emotionally dealing with a lot: I felt like I would never achieve my goals or reach my dreams or have a normal life because of my health, and that was immensely frustrating and upsetting.

It was what it was, and most of my friends from that era and I grew apart. I did have some great memories that will last a lifetime and will always think of them fondly, nonetheless. Luckily, when I transferred home from Clarion University and got off some medications, I eventually felt more like myself. I was out of an emotionally-abusive romantic relationship, loving my time at Pitt, and enjoying a part-time job and two great internships (one, as a proofreader at an advertising agency, and the other, on-air at 96.1 KISS FM with the awesome DJ Bonics.) But people didn't always understand. One close friend completely abandoned me for no reason;

another told me she was glad I had a good support system because she no longer chose to be a part of it. Those words cut like a knife, and to this day were one of the worst things that a person has ever said to me — particularly because they were when I was newly-diagnosed with celiac, still struggling with my RA and some other undiagnosed conditions, and needing close friendships the most.

I'm not perfect, so I forgive all of these people because I would hope that they, too, would forgive me and continue to love me through my shortcomings. People won't always understand what those of us who live with invisible (but chronic, lifelong, and incurable) health problems go through day-to-day, physically and emotionally. Sometimes, friendships and relationships end because it's our fault, and sometimes because it's someone else's. Often, though, the diseases that we live with play some kind of role in the demise of friendships and relationships — and we may not ever realize the full part they played until we are gifted with hindsight that's 20/20.

It's both upsetting and funny to see, from my perspective, how my illnesses inadvertently affect others. Once, while consumed with worry, my mom got hit in the head with a mechanical parking gate arm in the hospital parking garage. As we were leaving the hospital, she was distracted by my health situation and walked right into it as it closed down on her. It promptly knocked her on the ground, and I worried that we'd have to trudge right back on in to the hospital — me, newly-discharged, and she as the new patient. That's a funny (and very literal) example, but I know that she, my dad, my husband, grandparents, brother, and friends, all tend to worry about me now and then, whether they would admit it or not. That's a hard thing to handle for me: I hate being the reason for someone's else's worry, and I never want to burden those around me. It leads to a lot of guilt on my end, even though my circumstances are largely uncontrollable.

Luckily, I know that they don't hold it against me. I have a really strong group of friends these days who are endlessly supportive, uplifting, and encouraging. Some, I've known since childhood, others are brand-new. I feel completely and totally blessed to have them, as well as my loving husband and family, and even my pets (3 dogs: Lucy, Maggie, and Brutus; 2 cats: Jack-Jack and Theo; and 2 frogs: Kermie and Romeo.) All of that love is much-needed and much-appreciated throughout this always-difficult, never-predictable journey. I've also found great comfort in my church, and my volunteer work with the Arthritis Foundation and various other health and animal welfare organizations, including WearWoof, where I am the secretary on the Board of Directors. I also find great strength, support, inspiration, and encouragement through my online community via Arthritis Ashley, Ultimate You, and Rheum to Grow, and I have a lot of fun with my fashion and entertainment blog, Glitzburgh, too. Social media has afforded me so many opportunities, both personal and professional, and I am ever-grateful for the role it has played in shaping my life and helping me to positively affect the lives of others in addition to my own. If it weren't for MySpace, I wouldn't have reconnected with Mike, who is now my husband. Without Twitter, I wouldn't know Valerie, (ironically one of *two* close friends of mine named Val,) who has become one of the greatest and most dedicated friends I could ask for. Without Instagram, I may not have connected with my insta-BFF Hadley. Without AOL back in the day, I would have never met my "pen pal for life," Christina. And without Facebook, I probably wouldn't be able to talk with other sick people from all over the entire world who uplift me on a daily basis as I navigate this health journey right alongside them.

But with all of the sharing of education and information, and with all of the awareness, advocacy, inspiration, and motivation, comes some negativity, too. The amount of internet trolls and social media drama that I've encountered in recent years is nearly unfathomable. Just this past weekend, someone argued with me that celiac disease is not a real disease and that is a "first world problem" that only affects the privileged.

The night before my brain surgery, a guy called me a "pharma sheep" and told me, "good luck at the butcher." (Classy.)

Last year, I would get messages from an anonymous profile telling me how ugly I was, that I looked like Bugs Bunny, that "fat bald Britney Spears" was hotter than I'd ever hope be, that no one cares about my life, that my blogs are stupid, I'm pathetic, and so on. I've had people tell me that I'm not really sick. I've had people completely bash me and rip me apart for talking about my experiences with natural treatments, and I've had people throw shade at me for even discussing my health problems at all. Then, there are the folks who think that being sick is some kind of contest. They turn every post into a "who is sicker" competition, turning commiserating into sheer misery. The bitterness and toxicity that radiates off of my computer screen is absolutely jarring sometimes.

I realize that life with illness isn't pleasant or fun, but there's really no point in taking it out on other people. I am always open, real, and honest, but while I strive to do it, I don't think that it is humanly possible to be entirely positive all the time — especially while dealing with health problems. However, I don't believe that there is ever any excuse to be unkind or cruel towards others. We should be lifting one another up, not tearing each other down.

I won't judge you for your choices if you don't judge me for mine. You may not agree with my choices, and that's okay. For example, I have tattoos — currently, 5 of them. At present, I have hues of pink in my blond (but naturally almost Kardashian-level brunette) hair. I'm certainly Christian, but I like and respect various life principles and values found in other religions — and I'm into science, too. I don't see why these things need to be mutually exclusive, or why they cannot coexist. I am now vegetarian — mostly vegan, in fact. But, even though I hope to stay on the proverbial meatless wagon, I may not always be able to do so. As aforementioned — I'm not perfect. (Plus, I am a recovering bacon-a-holic, after all.) I am a mix of Carrie Bradshaw and Charlotte York. I'm equal parts "basic" and "hipster." I'm half Holly Golightly and half Gwen Stefani. I used to be really conservative in my political views; now I'm much more liberal. (But I'm basically right down the middle, if we're being honest.) So, whether it is my appearance, my faith, or my points of view about health, I don't fit neatly into any kind of little box — nor would I ever want to.

But, here's the thing: it's not anyone's place to judge me for that. Only God can judge me, and that's a notion that I'll stand by. People attacking me for being myself, for trying to help others, or for sharing my medical journey is absolutely frustrating and disheartening. People ignorantly arguing with me regarding actual facts is even more maddening.

They do say, though, that your haters are among your biggest fans. So I hope that my trolls at least bought a copy of this book — even if they'll undoubtedly burn it and then write a one-star negative review on Amazon to follow.

THAT TIME I MET *NSYNC AND YEARS LATER FINISHED A HEALTH MEMOIR

My illnesses have thrown me for many a loop, personally, professionally, and emotionally. In a lot of ways, my health problems have in part shaped who I am, while simultaneously robbing me of being as "me" as I'd like to be. There are little things that we sickies have to occasionally give up: nights out with friends, certain kinds of shoes, sunbathing, sports, wheat. There are big things that some of us have had to sacrifice or modify, too, because of illness. Some of us have had to change career goals or end relationships. Some have gone through depression, or gained weight. There are some people with rheumatoid arthritis, lupus, and other chronic conditions who have lost way worse: the ability to walk, limbs, babies, and, for some, even their lives. Those are sad realities that we cannot forget. Those are sad realities that many people in the general public don't even know about — or, if they do, that they may not want to face. I am grateful, despite living for most of my life with health problems, that I've not had to use a wheelchair other than in the hospital (and that one time at the airport,) and that I still had a nice

153

childhood and fun teenage experience despite being ill. I am grateful that in the midst of sickness I've still been able to achieve some cool things, and I'm thankful that I possess some treasured memories and awesome life experiences in spite of it. Not everyone is as fortunate, sick or not — and I never forget that.

So, in the grand scheme of things, the little minor instances that I've had to modify or miss out on in life are just that: minor. Sure, I've sat out of softball games or gym classes, and regularly have to cancel plans with friends. No, I'll probably never be a runner like I sometimes am in my dreams at night. Yes, I've had some bad experiences with past employers. I've missed out on concerts because of everything from brain surgery to strep throat, and I've had to give up my love for high heels and cute, sexy stilettos. I'll probably never have the kind of body I want — either appearance-wise or health-wise. My legs are ugly, my knee is deformed. My hair has thinned; I'm sometimes puffy from medications. I'm now allergic to just about everything on earth, and it isn't abnormal to see an old hospital bracelet in my garbage can, or the gummy remains of a bandage in the crook of my elbow from where I had blood drawn. I'll probably never play softball again. Badly limping around the Magic Kingdom was a disappointing, yet expected, part of a recent Disney trip. Ordering at a restaurant will always cause me a moment of trepidation. After a vacation or a busy weekend, my body will always need a day or two to recover. The flu could set me back a whole month or two. I'll end a lot of sentences with "…as long as I feel okay," and I'll have to cancel plans more than

I'd like to. I'll never be a perfect housewife or the friend who's always available to hang out at the drop of a hat.

But despite all of those things that my health problems have taken away from me, they've given me some gifts along the way, too. I'm strong. I now am more loving, compassionate, and empathetic towards others. I always try to be kind and respectful, and I try not to judge, because I don't know what others are going through privately. I would expect that people do the same towards me, though I have learned that many will not. I have learned to not jump to conclusions, though. After all, some people are dealing with things we are unaware of — maybe health-related, maybe not. Look at me and millions of others like me: at first glance, you wouldn't think we were ill. However, what we see is not always what we get. Life is full of surprises, and people are full of them, too. I've learned to try to stress less about inconsequential matters, because some people have really big, life-altering issues that they're dealing with. I know, because I've been there myself. So I try to keep perspective. My health problems are a lot worse than most people I know, this is true. Then again, I know people who have it way worse than me, also. This is a good reminder that when things are bad, they could always be worse. Everyone has his or her own burdens and problems — mine just happen to be health-related. I'm blessed in other areas where other people may not be, and I know that. My health problems have taught me to always focus on the good instead of the bad, to find humor in every situation, and to remain strong in my faith and steadfast in my mission of healing. I've learned to be a steward of my health, and to invest in it wisely. Investing in my body now seems more important than going to every concert or buying every new shade of OPI nail polish or every new album that drops, like I used to do. Suddenly, it makes more sense to spend money on supplements or medicinal treatments instead of handbags and clothing and martinis. So I've been learning patience, too. Right now, maybe I do have to focus more on my health than I'd like to — but I'm doing it so that hopefully in the future, I can focus on bigger and brighter things. It may not be this way forever, but it may. I have accepted that, too.

I try to surround myself with people who are the mirrors that reflect my own values of love and light. I want to see God in people; I want to see love and compassion, laughter and smiles, empathy and happiness, positivity and good. I want to feel good vibes. I want to be a prayer in action. I want to nurture a kind heart in myself and to bring out those kind hearts in others. I want to commiserate with fellow chronic illness warriors who are striving to thrive, who are focused on healing, who want to live in the light and not dwell in the dark. I want to bring that light to those who are hurting.

But, I try not to surround myself with those who are bitter, negative, or otherwise toxic. I want to help them, but I have learned to love these types of people from a distance. I am a true empath whose energy feeds off those around me. When it comes to emotions, I can literally almost feel what other people are feeling. If you bring too much anxiety, stress, melancholy, or negativity to the table, I find it stressful to be around you, and I feel it on a nearly physical level. It's nothing personal: it's just the energy.

This could be physical or even conveyed online. I carry your burden whether I want to or not — and that can be a challenge when I already have my own cross to bear on top of it. To be around negativity on a consistent basis drains me in a quite tangible way, and so, sometimes, I have to even take a step back from people close to me or from the online chronic illness community. I'm sure some of you can relate.

I just feel that there's no use in making myself sicker due to unwarranted stress and unnecessary drama, online or otherwise. I don't want to hear petty complaints about first-world problems. I need to concentrate on finding the good parts of this crappy situation instead of focusing on the bad ones. I don't want to let my health problems - or other people - bring me down in any way, and I would encourage that you do the same. There's nothing wrong with distancing yourself from people or situations that bring negativity or toxicity to your life. You have enough to deal with healthwise, you shouldn't have to deal with uncalled-for bad vibes in addition to that. It isn't selfish or indulgent to practice self-care. It shouldn't be a luxury to take care of and nurture your body. It's not opulence: it's crucial to your survival, and I'd urge you all to remember that.

My health — or lack thereof — has given me a kind of inner strength, grace, and serenity that I lacked for so many years. Even just five or six short years ago, I was far more negative, far more bitter, and far less hopeful. Now, I feel focused, calm, and at peace. I'm not always happy about my health — in fact, sometimes, I get really mad, sad, and frustrated. I have my Sick Idiot nutties and my mega-breakdowns now and then. But, I try to handle myself with grace and with fortitude. I have been tested a lot in my life and I will surely continue to be tested even more, as will all of you.

But I thank God all the time for my mental toughness, my empath's heart, and my motivation and determination to get what I want despite my circumstances.

I think back to a time in high school when I was utterly, unwaveringly determined to meet the popular boy band *NSync. My mom thought I was insane as I dragged my friend Caroline downtown on the bus. I had a tip about which hotel they may be staying at, and I knew it in my heart of hearts that it was going to happen. It was as though I willed it into existence when the five guys — including my love, Justin Timberlake — waltzed out moments later, making their way to their car. A couple of them (JC Chasez and Lance Bass, to be precise) stopped for photos, and it made for a fun story that we'll tell for years to come. (It should also be noted that Justin Timberlake waved to me that day, and 12 years later would also say hello to me — with eye contact! — when I introduced myself to him in NYC. I realize that mentioning this is total not-so-humble-bragging, but ... come on. It's Justin Timberlake. It's warranted. Also: I say that these encounters count as meeting him, but my husband does not concur. This disagreement caused quite a heated family-wide debate one Christmas Eve.)

That *NSync occurrence, though, as odd as it seems, is a sort of metaphor for my life. It sounded crazy — and it was crazy — but, just like I knew it in my heart of hearts that I could go see Oprah one day, or raise thousands of dollars for charity while being in and out of the hospital — I simply knew I could meet them if I set my mind to it, even when others didn't believe me. And after the fact, even though it obviously happened and I had photo proof, kids at school still didn't believe me that it really occurred. That's how life with illness is, too — I could produce medical records and x-rays and MRI scans and biopsies and all the rest, and some people will still never believe me, despite the proof. Some people will never understand — or, perhaps, maybe it's that some people will never want to even *try* to understand.

Like the great *NSync Meeting of 2001, I believe that I will overcome my health problems — and if I don't, I believe that I can still live a full, happy, thriving life, nonetheless. That may sound crazy, but I know it to be true. I'm a Sick Idiot, but I'm a Sick Idiot who can overcome great things and get over great barriers when I put my mind to it.

So can you.

AFTERTHOUGHTS AND
THE INSPIRATIONAL STUFF

Just in the last month alone, I've been at the hospital twice, had to get an MRI because of a "Chiari scare," and have had my fair share of injections and IVs. I also had a bad sinus infection that lasted 2 months and wouldn't respond to antibiotics. I've had to temporarily stop exercising until I see a cardiologist. I've had to explain my Enbrel syringe to a TSA agent when I was traveling to the beach. Chest pain, elbow pain and back pain have been prominent as of late. It would be easy to get down about it all, and at times, I have. I am human. I have had a couple of moments of weakness lately where I've gotten really angry about my situation, but then I realized that it's okay. It's hard, but it's okay. I've accomplished a lot despite my health.

In fact, I've done more even while being sick than some of my healthier peers have done while being healthy — and while it isn't a competition, that means something to me personally. When you always feel different, and have at times even felt "less than" because of your health problems, any little achievement big or small feels like something really special. And it is. So I try not to let my physical difficulties consume or define me. That said, I know things could be worse, but at the same time, if I'm being honest, it still isn't easy. I don't want to portray an unrealistic sense that it is.

To be clear, barely any of the issues that I've mentioned throughout this book have been resolved, even to this day. There are even other ailments I've been diagnosed with that I haven't made much mention of in this collection of stories — but they still contribute to the cornucopia of symptoms that I experience almost daily. Nearly every time that I've thought I've found a treatment or a fix, it has failed. I thought brain surgery would be the answer to my prayers, and while it helped some things, it certainly wasn't the miracle I'd been hoping for. The same rings true for many medications, for the gluten-free diet, and so on. For the most part, I still struggle — and often struggle even more year after year. At 31 years old, I still have little-to-no answers. Often, I feel like I am on an unresolved episode of *Mystery Diagnosis*. My husband and I joke that I have a yet-unnamed autoimmune disease that is exclusive to me, and, apparently, me only.

If it wasn't for my goal to try to find something good in every day, I wouldn't be able to function nearly as well as I do. It would be easy to give up and to be a persistent pessimist or a Debbie Downer. That's the easy way out. The easy way is to give in to the excruciating pain, or to let the overwhelming sickness and unrelenting fatigue win.

But what fun would life be if we always took the easy route? What good would it do us to stay confined within our comfort zones? How can we flourish and grow if we are content to remain a victim of our own mindsets? We may not be able to control the fact that, at times, or bodies feel like some version of a prison or purgatory. We can, however, control our attitude in any situation. We can always choose how we respond to our circumstances. We can decide whether we are going to be bitter and dwell on the negative aspects of life, or, if we are going to try to be positive and happy despite our struggles. We can make our mess our message, turn our burdens into blessings, and our pain into power. We can be overcomers if we allow ourselves to be. We didn't choose our situations, but we can choose who we become in spite of them.

Or, we can simply waste our days complaining, becoming content in the not-doing. After all, the not-doing is easy. The complaining is easy. What's difficult is to make that choice to be positive or happy, and to try to be productive or fulfilled, even when the rational thing to do is to be sad or apathetic. What's hard is to get up out of bed each morning and make the best of a crappy situation, when no one would blame you if you just gave up. That's what's hard.

I recall last summer when I spoke at a Juvenile Arthritis Family Day event presented by the Arthritis Foundation here in Pittsburgh. It had been my second time speaking on stage at such an occasion, and, for some reason, this time I felt even more empowered than I ever had before. The first time, I shared my story but had not yet had as many life experiences to point out. I was not at a place personally where I could say to these kids, "LOOK! You can do it, despite being sick! You can accomplish things, even if you have juvenile arthritis or another illness." The second time I spoke at JA Family Day, though, I felt more confident in sharing my journey — because I felt that I truly had something to show for myself other than the label of "patient." I felt that, even though I was still in the trenches right alongside them, a part of me had learned to thrive despite my circumstances. I felt moved, because I felt like, for the first time, that my pain had a purpose. Perhaps this life of illness was given to me because I was strong enough to handle it, and would able to use it for good. Or, perhaps, it was luck of the draw, and purely random. The truth is, it doesn't matter. I got the diagnoses I got, and I was dealt the cards of life that I was dealt. It doesn't matter what caused my illnesses, why this has happened to me, or even which condition came first. It doesn't matter which is the primary diagnosis, or if some of the diagnoses are inaccurate, because, to me, all that matters is how I respond to my situation and how I choose to live my life in spite of it. It is about moving forward.

It is frustrating to me that some people don't believe in the severity of these illnesses. It is maddening that there are still some folks out there who mistakenly believe that RA is "just arthritis," or celiac is "just a sensitivity," or migraines are "just headaches," or that I'm "too young" for this stuff. But, as frustrating and maddening as those things can be, it doesn't matter. It doesn't matter if we call it rheumatoid arthritis or autoimmune arthritis or rheumatoid disease. It doesn't matter if we choose to take a holistic approach or a traditional one. What matters, in my mind, are the following three things:

1. **That we live our own life as best we can.** Stay in your lane and focus on your own journey — don't compete with or compare yourself to others. There is no right or wrong way to be sick.

2. **That we strive to spread awareness.** You may not be a lobbying-on-Capitol Hill activist or an online powerhouse when it comes to advocacy and awareness, but even educating your closest friends and family makes a difference in the long run.

3. **That we are stewards of our own health.** This means that you must take responsibility for your own health. Be your own advocate. Educate yourself. Try your very best to be as healthy as you can despite your circumstances. Take good care of your body. Try. Realize that it matters. You have a responsibility to not give up — you owe it to yourselves and to others who you may inspire every day without even knowing it.

If you can do these things, and strive to focus on gratitude, grace, and humor, I think that you can still live a full, happy, and even relatively healthy life despite being handed a medical diagnosis *(or, almost 40 of them. But who's counting?)*

After all, even a Sick Idiot day is a good day to be alive.

THE END

GLOSSARY:
SOME MEDICAL CONDITIONS EXPLAINED

Here, I will explain some of my more prominent diagnoses.

Celiac Disease a.k.a. Coeliac disease, Celiac Sprue, or Gluten Enteropathy: Celiac disease is a genetic autoimmune disorder that mostly affects the small intestine, though it may have neurological implications, as well. In people with celiac, simply ingesting certain offending proteins containing an amino-acid sequence collectively known as gluten will set off an immune-system response that causes a quantifiable level of damage to the patient's small intestine. This inflammatory response is quite destructive and interferes with the body's ability to properly absorb vitamins, minerals, and nutrients from food. This leads to malnutrition and a host of other systemic symptoms and complications. Celiac feels like you have a hangover, all the time, sometimes coupled with food poisoning and an allergy attack on top of it when you get "glutened." Wheat: it's what's <u>not</u> for dinner.

Chiari Malformation a.k.a. Arnold-Chiari Malformation: A Chiari malformation is a structural defect in the cerebellum, which is the part of the brain that controls a person's balance. In short, it is a brain herniation. Symptoms of this disorder of the brain may include, but are not limited to, neck pain, balance problems, muscle weakness, numbness and tingling, difficulty swallowing, headache, fatigue, facial pain, ringing in the ears, hearing loss, vomiting, insomnia, brain fog, and paralysis. Sometimes, hand coordination and fine motor skills may also be affected. Chiari feels like the back of your head is going to explode at any given moment. The additional widespread body pain and often-vague neurological symptoms are frightening and frustrating. Chiarians are often known as "zipperheads" because of our unique scars post-surgery.

Chronic Migraine: Chronic migraine is a part of the spectrum of migraine disorders. Qualifying to be diagnosed with chronic migraine means that a patient has a headache on 15 days or more per month for 3 or more months, of which 8 or more days meet the medical criteria for being a migraine. A migraine is a complex neurological condition with a wide variety of symptoms. For many people, the main feature is a grueling headache, often accompanied with nausea, vomiting, visual disturbances, neck and facial pain, and fatigue — but migraines can present themselves in a variety of ways. The manifestation of a migraine may vary from patient to patient. Migraines can be exceedingly disabling, and are often debilitating to the point of affecting a person's quality of life and having a major impact on employability and more. To me, a migraine feels like my head is going to explode while my eyes bulge out of their sockets like a cartoon character and I throw up my gluten-free lunch everywhere. There have been times where I've experienced vice-grip-level migraines and thought, *"A lobotomy would be nice right about now."*

Lupus a.k.a. SLE or systemic lupus erythematosus:
Lupus is a chronic inflammatory disease that occurs when your body's immune system attacks its own tissues and organs. As with RA, inflammation from lupus can affect many different body systems — including the joints, skin, kidneys, blood cells, brain, heart, and lungs. A malar facial rash, known as a butterfly rash, is a hallmark symptom. Lupus feels as though you are dealing with hot flashes and facial rashes on top of an RA and Celiac flare combined. For me, the fatigue associated with a lupus flare is the most intense fatigue of all. Butterflies are pretty, but we lupus butterflies are pretty badass, too.

Rheumatoid Arthritis a.k.a. RA, rheumatoid disease, or autoimmune arthritis: Not just for old people, rheumatoid arthritis, unlike osteoarthritis, is a systemic inflammatory autoimmune disease that manifests itself in multiple joints of the body and can affect people at basically any age. The inflammatory process mostly affects the lining of the joints called synovium, but can also attack other major organs of the body. On an average day, RA feels like a mix between a sports injury (in multiple joints) coupled with the full-body ache, general sickness, and debilitating fatigue that come along with the flu. On a particularly bad day, it feels as though someone is pulling you apart at the joints, and then lighting the joint space on fire, while stabbing it at the same time. I kid you not. It's flippin' miserable, dude.

Sjögren's Syndrome: Sjögren's syndrome is a chronic autoimmune condition that is generally characterized by a primary deterioration of the salivary and lachrymal glands. This causes dryness in the patient's mouth, eyes, and other moisture-producing areas. It often accompanies other rheumatic immune system disorders like rheumatoid arthritis and lupus. Dry eyes and dry mouth are mainstays of the condition, but Sjögren's, much like the others, is a systemic disease. The symptoms may be felt throughout the entire body. With Sjögren's, my contacts bother me, my eyes feel dry, my mouth feels cottony, my lips get chapped, and my hair and fingernails sometimes hurt. I also don't sweat a lot even after intense cardio workouts. When I do sweat, however, I like to say, "I don't sweat, I sparkle."

Those are the main culprits, for me personally. If you're curious about any of the other diagnoses that I listed at the beginning, I encourage you to do some research on your own. You may be surprised what you can learn about this complex and expansive world of invisible chronic illness and autoimmune disease. I know that even I continue to discover more about it all each and every day.

GET INVOLVED

A portion of proceeds from Sick Idiot book sales will go to some of my personal favorite charities. Learn more about these conditions and how to donate, volunteer, or advocate by visiting their websites below:

- The Arthritis Foundation: www.arthritis.org

- The Lupus Foundation of America: www.lupus.org

- The National Foundation for Celiac Awareness: www.celiaccentral.org

- The Chiari and Syringomyelia Foundation: www.csfinfo.org

- The Sjögren's Syndrome Foundation: www.sjogrens.org

- The American Migraine Foundation: www.americanmigrainefoundation.org

- The American Autoimmune Related Diseases Association: www.aarda.org

- Stand Up to Cancer: www.standup2cancer.org

- The Leukemia & Lymphoma Society: www.lls.org

- The Children's Hospital of Pittsburgh Foundation: www.givetochildrens.org

Share your funniest or most inspiring **#SickIdiot** moments by using hashtag **#SickIdiot** on social media!

ABOUT THE AUTHOR

Ashley Boynes-Shuck is a writer, health coach, public speaker, and advocate based out of Pittsburgh, PA, where she lives with her husband and (many) pets. She has been writing for as long as she can remember. Ashley is the author of a fiction novel called *To Exist* and is known in the online chronic illness community as Arthritis Ashley. Her passions include reading, writing, animals, wellness, fashion, volunteering, and helping others. Through her advocacy and writing work, she hopes to uplift and inspire young people living with health problems. You can learn more by visiting her websites abshuck.com and ArthritisAshley.com. Tweet her at @abshuck or @ArthritisAshley.

TO EXIST

Ashley's debut fiction novel *To Exist* is the post-apocalyptic story of Shelby Weiss, a young breast cancer survivor and screenwriter who is believed to be the last woman left on earth. Join Shelby in her fight to survive as she struggles to exist while being hunted in this strange new world. Will she escape with her sanity and her health intact? Find out by ordering *To Exist* on amazon.com, BarnesAndNoble.com, or abshuck.com.

Also available as an e-book on Kindle and Nook.

23643857R00116

Made in the USA
Middletown, DE
02 September 2015